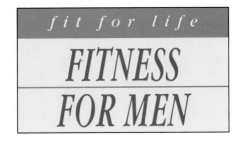

fit for life

FITNESS
FOR MEN

Credits:

Art Director: Peter Bridgewater
Editorial Consultants: Maria Pal/Clark Robinson Ltd
Photography: Paul Forrester, assisted by John Alflatt
Model: Steven Berrisford

Picture credits:

key: a = above; b = below

The author and publishers have made every effort to identify the
copyright owners of the photographs; they apologize for any
omissions and wish to thank the following:

Sheila Buff, 82/83; Paul J. Sutton, 78/79; Trevor Wood, 6/7, 68/69,
77, 81, 85.

They would also like to thank Reebok International Limited for
supplying props for photography, and the Gatwick Hilton
International.

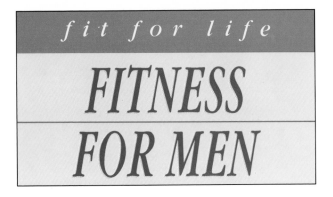

fit for life

FITNESS
FOR MEN

BRUCE BYRON

Gallery Books
an imprint of W.H. Smith Publishers, Inc.
112 Madison Avenue, New York
New York 10016

A QUARTO BOOK

This edition published in 1990 by Gallery Books,
an imprint of W.H. Smith Publishers, Inc.,
112, Madison Avenue, New York, New York 10016

Gallery Books are available for bulk purchase for
sales promotions and premium use. For details write or
telephone the Manager of Special Sales, W.H. Smith
Publishers Inc., 112 Madison Avenue, New York, New
York 10016. (212) 532-6600.

ISBN 0-8317-3893-6

The information and recommendations contained in this book
are intended to complement, not substitute for, the advice of
your own physician. Before starting any medical treatment,
exercise program or diet, consult your physician. Information is
given without any guarantees on the part of the author and
publisher, and they cannot be held responsible for the contents
of this book.

► CONTENTS

▶ *INTRODUCTION TO FITNESS*

In today's fast-paced world you have to be in good shape to keep up with everyone else. Exercise and a healthy diet will enable you to enjoy life with vitality and zest.

Many people have the misconception that the only way to exercise is to workout at a health club. Although a health club gives you an incentive to exercise just because everyone around you is straining and sweating, you can workout anywhere! At home, in the office, even on a business trip, there's always a time and a place for exercise.

Our plan is to give you some basic exercises that will make you fit. Special attention will be paid to problem areas like the waist and stomach. The relatively new program known as aerobics will be explored, teaching you the standard high-impact exercises as well as the revolutionary low-impact methods.

Proper workouts will also strengthen your muscles, making them less susceptible to injury. We'll cover a wide range of warm-up drills designed to keep you injury-free during your workouts. A

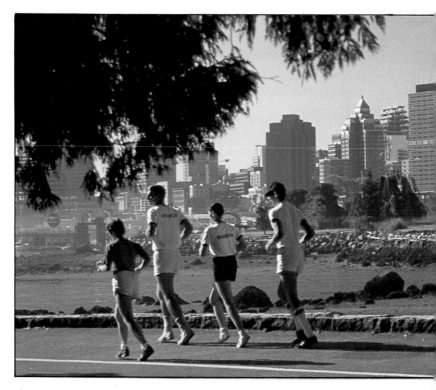

special section will teach you exercises to avoid those awfully painful backaches.

Almost all of our exercises require no additional equipment other than proper work-out clothes and shoes. We'll even show you how to select the proper shoes to keep your feet hopping and jumping. The few exercises that require weights are structured so that you can use any five-pound object around the home. There's no need to purchase expensive barbell equipment. Our goal is to make your workout simple, easy, and efficient. The more enjoyable your exercise routine, the more likely you are to stick with it.

Since almost all of us play some sort of sport, we'll show you ways to increase your endurance and strength geared toward the dynamics of the sport. You'll be able to incorporate most of our beginning exercises to build your body for the demands of your favorite sport.

So if you want to get that bounce and zoom into every step, break out the sweatpants and sneakers and let's get fit!

Jogging is one of the most convenient and sociable ways of building up basic fitness. The only additional equipment you'll need are good shoes to absorb the pressure if you run any distances on hard sidewalks or streets.

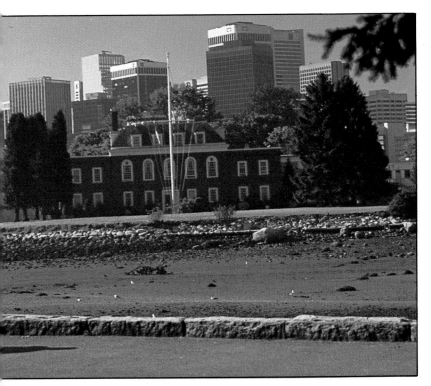

▶ *TORSO WARM-UPS*

Many of us who do any warm-ups before exercises or athletic events concentrate just on the arms and legs. Although its true that these limbs seem to suffer the most injuries, the torso, particularly the stomach and back, can also be damaged. So let's warm-up the main core of the body with some simple torso exercises.

SIDE BENDS

Stand erect, spread your feet apart, and keep your hands at sides.

Bend sideways to the right until your right hand is touching your upper thigh and then slowly return to starting position.

Repeat on the left side. Keep the back straight at all times. Do 10 repetitions (10×) on each side.

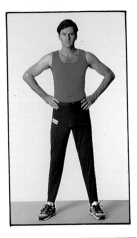

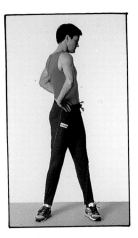

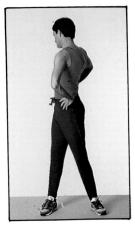

TRUNK TURNS

Stand erect, spread your feet apart and keep hands at hips.

Keeping the back straight, twist your body so that your right elbow is facing the same direction as your toes.

Return to the starting position and repeat, this time twisting the other way. Do 10× on each side.

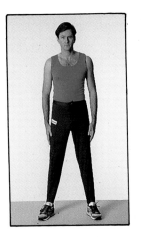

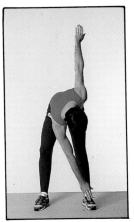

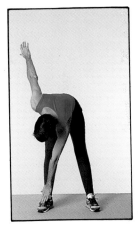

TOE TOUCHES

Stand erect with your feet apart.

Hold your arms up above your head and reach down with your right hand and touch your left foot or ankle.

Return to the starting position and then repeat with the left hand on right foot or ankle. Do 10×.

9

▶ HEAD AND SHOULDERS WARM-UPS

Too many of us ignore exercising the head, neck and shoulder areas. Since most sports require quick responses and eye–hand coordination, many times a snap of the head results in a pulled muscle. So if you really want to be able to put your nose to the grindstone and excel at your sport, let's warm up the head and shoulders!

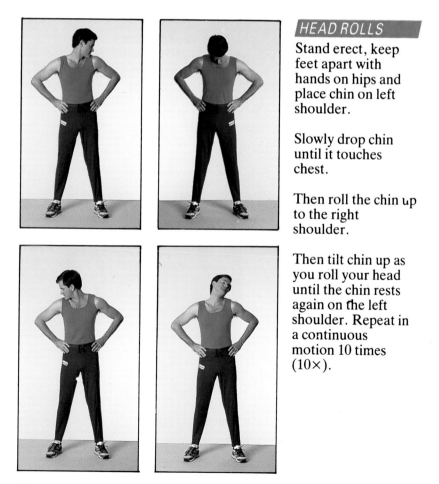

HEAD ROLLS

Stand erect, keep feet apart with hands on hips and place chin on left shoulder.

Slowly drop chin until it touches chest.

Then roll the chin up to the right shoulder.

Then tilt chin up as you roll your head until the chin rests again on the left shoulder. Repeat in a continuous motion 10 times (10×).

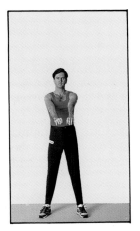

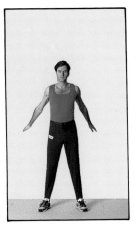

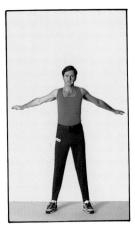

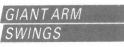

GIANT ARM SWINGS

Stand erect with arms held straight up above the head and drop them slowly in a swinging motion in front of your body.

Continue the motion, bringing your arms past your body.

Complete the movement by swinging arms back up to the starting position. Repeat in a continuous motion 10×.

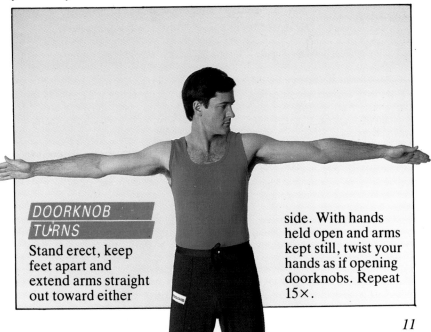

DOORKNOB TURNS

Stand erect, keep feet apart and extend arms straight out toward either side. With hands held open and arms kept still, twist your hands as if opening doorknobs. Repeat 15×.

▶ *THIGH WARM-UPS*

Any athletic event that includes leaping and jumping requires you to have well-developed thighs. The thighs provide the power with which you can propel your body off the floor. When you drive your legs up getting ready to spike that volleyball, the springing motion starts with the thighs. Here are a few good exercises to warm up and develop your upper leg muscles. Try them on for thighs!

LUNGES

Stand erect. Keep feet apart and hands on hips. Turn your right foot outward. Bend or lunge toward the right, dipping your body and keeping your left leg straight. Return to starting position and then repeat lunging toward the left. Repeat 10 times (10×) on either side.

HALF-SQUATS

Stand erect. Keep feet apart and hands on hips. With knees and legs slightly turned out, dip down six inches and hold for three seconds. Return to starting position. Repeat 10×.

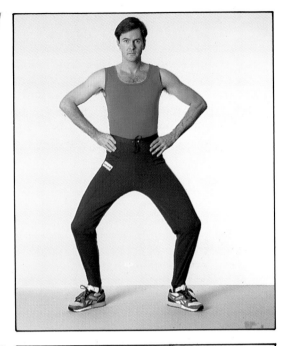

HURDLE STRETCHES

Sit on floor with left leg straight ahead and right leg bent at the knee. Your right ankle should be touching your buttocks. Reach out with your arms and grab your left ankle. Hold for three seconds. Release and return to starting position. Then extend right leg, bend left leg at knee and repeat. Do 8× on each leg.

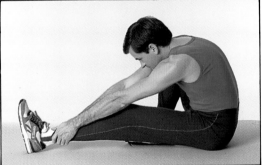

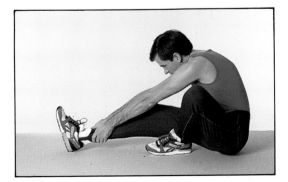

▶ *LEG WARM-UPS*

Every exercise and sport, including swimming, relies on a set of strong legs. Running, jumping, lunging, and squatting requires you to have powerful legs for success. The legs are also prone to injury, so any proper warm-up must include a number of leg exercises. Using these exercises will help you get a leg up on the competition!

CALF STRETCHES

Stand about a foot away from a wall, a tree, or the like. Keep your feet slightly spread and lean forward. Support your weight with your hands, keeping your back straight. Make sure your heels are pressing into the ground. Hold for three seconds and then return to starting position. Repeat 5×.

CALF RAISES

Stand erect with your toes on the edge of a block of wood, a book, or the like. Keep your back straight and your arms at your sides. Raise the body, swinging your arms forward until you are standing on your toes. Hold for three seconds and return to starting position. Repeat 10×.

KNEE CLASPS

Sit on the floor with your legs extended.

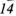

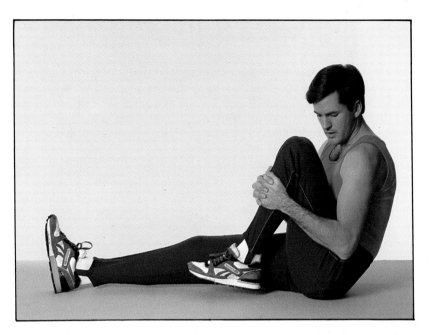

Pull your left knee up until it touches the chest. At the same time clasp your hands around the left knee. Hold briefly.

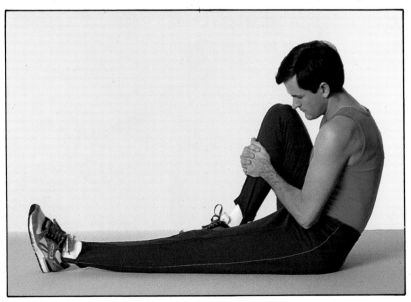

Release knee, return to the starting position and repeat with the right knee. Do 10 repetitions (10×).

▶ *BASIC WARM-UP ROUTINE*

Like any other machine, the body has to be warmed up before it can operate properly. If you've ever started a car on a cold morning, you know how cranky the engine becomes if you don't take the time to let the engine's lubricants and parts warm up. Your body's tissues and circulation also needs to be primed for action before you throw them into gear!

Watch any professional athlete. From baseball to swimming, they all take the time to stretch and warm up their muscles. For some sports, like basketball and tennis, you need to spend a few minutes taking practice shots, just to get the movement of the game in mind. Do you really think a professional football player needs to practice catching passes minutes before the game? That player has been catching footballs since grade school. But he takes the time to run out and catch a few because those muscles may not be the same ones he exercised in the pre-game weight room. Professional athletes know that the better your body is warmed up, the less likely you are to be injured and the more responsive your muscles will be.

For your exercise program, we've incorporated some of the basic routines discussed earlier in the book. Besides this warm-up, you should check the section dealing with any specific sports you may play. Remember to take your time warming up and your body will thank you with fitness and vitality.

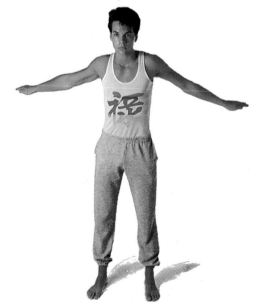

WARM-UP ROUTINE

- Side Bends — five on each side.
- Trunk Turns — five on each side.
- Toe Touches — 10 on each side.
- Head Rolls — five in each direction.
- Shoulder Shrugs — five times.
- The Reach — five times on each side.
- Waist Twists — five on each side.
- The Punch — 10 on each side.
- Chest Pulls (1 or 2) — five times.
- The Deep Breath — three times.
- Basic Jog — two minutes.

▶ *BREATH SAVERS*

Many times during your workout, the body will be crying out for a brief rest. Since you're getting warmed-up, it would be counter-productive to stop now. Here are a few exercises that give you a chance to catch your breath and still continue the workout.

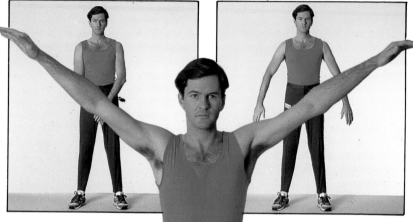

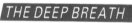

THE DEEP BREATH

Stand erect with your feet apart, your hands crossed in front of your groin and your arms fully extended.

Take a deep breath as you swing your arms out to either side.

Continue the motion until your hands meet above your head and hold for three seconds.

Then slowly return to the starting position as you exhale. Repeat 5×.

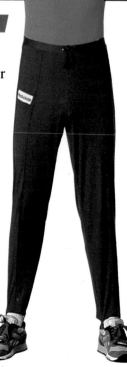

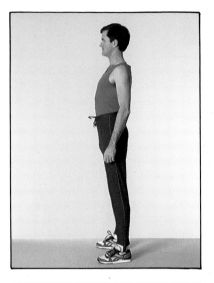

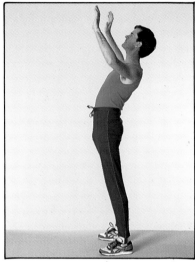

THE REACH

Stand erect, keep your feet apart and your hands loosely at your sides.

Take a long, deep breath as you slowly bend backward, pushing your hips forward at the same time as raising your arms.

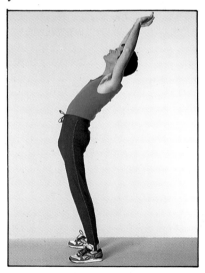

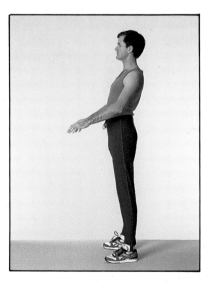

Reach upward with your fingers extended toward the ceiling above your head and hold for three seconds.

Then slowly return to the starting position as you exhale. Do 5 repetitions (5×).

▶ *WASTE THE WAIST*

The waist is always the toughest part of the body to keep fit. Since it is only used in twisting motions, most of us never fully exercise that area of the body. Soon "love handles" and "flab flaps" develop, causing us to seek ways to waste the waist. Here are a few exercises to deal with those waisty matters.

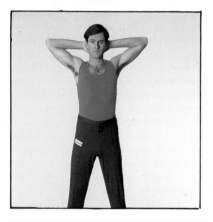

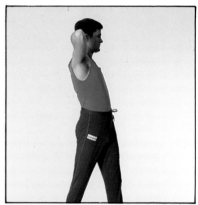

WAIST TWISTS

Stand erect with your feet apart and your hands clasped behind your head.

Hold your stomach in and slowly twist your body to the left.

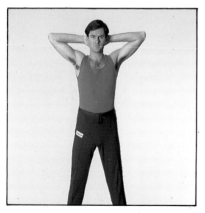

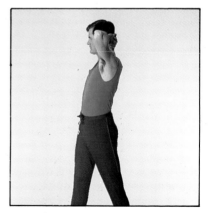

Keeping your back straight, return to the starting position.

Repeat by twisting to the right. Do 10 repetitions (10×) on each side.

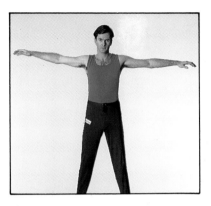

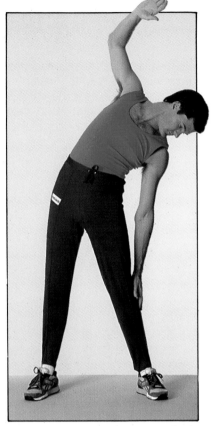

WAIST LEANS

Stand erect. Keep your feet apart with your arms extended out on either side.
Lean down toward the left until your hand touches the outer side of your left knee.
Return to the starting position and repeat with the right hand. Do 10× on each side.

WAIST TILTS

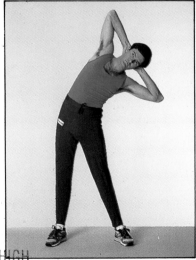

Stand erect with your feet apart and your hands clasped behind your head.

Hold your stomach in and slowly tilt your upper body so that your left elbow bends toward your hip.

Keep your back straight to prevent you from leaning forward, return to the starting position and repeat by tilting to the right side. Do 10× on each side.

▶ *BELLY BURNERS*

We'd all love to have firm, flat stomachs. A strong abdomen is a great way to prevent lower back strain, since it helps to prevent stress during lifting and bending. The only way to get that stomach fit is through a continual effort and workout with these belly burners.

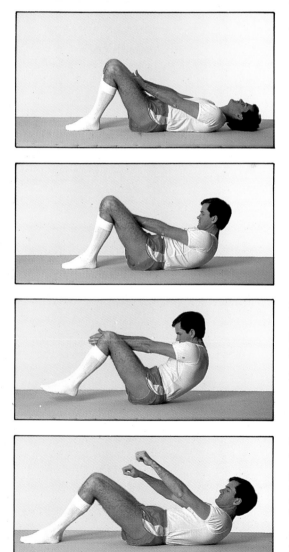

CRUNCHES

Lie on the floor with your legs about eight inches apart and bend your legs at the knees so that your feet are flat on the ground.

Extend your hands through your knees and clasp your hands together while tucking your chin down near your chest.

Slowly, while tightening the stomach, raise your shoulders off the ground as you reach through your knees.

Once you are about three inches off the ground, drop back down to the starting position. Do not bounce, but instead drop slowly. Do 30 repetitions (30×).

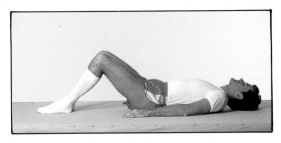

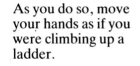

CLIMB THE LADDER

Lie on the floor with your legs about eight inches apart and bend your legs so that your feet are flat on the ground.

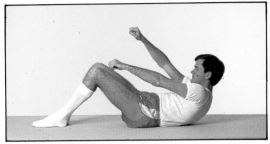

Extend your hands above the knees, tuck in your stomach and slowly begin to raise off the ground.

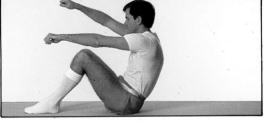

As you do so, move your hands as if you were climbing up a ladder.

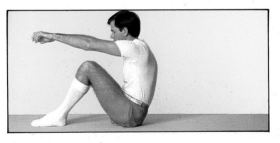

Complete the movement until you've pulled your chest up to your knees.

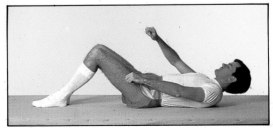

Then climb back down the ladder until you're back to the starting position. Repeat 20×.

▶ *WAIST STRETCHERS*

Since keeping the waist thin and trim is such a difficult chore, here are some advanced exercises to attack that excess flab. One way to reduce the extra baggage is to make the waist area more flexible and to increase the elasticity. Try these workouts to stretch the waist.

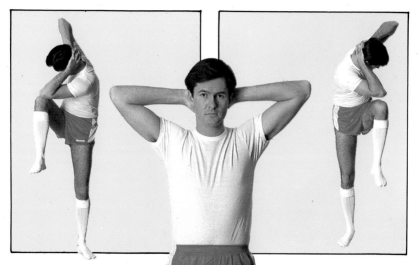

KNEE GRINDS

Stand erect with your feet apart and your hands clasped behind head.

Bring your right knee up and touch it with your descending left elbow.

Return to starting position and then bring your left knee up and touch it with your right elbow. Do 10 repetitions (10×).

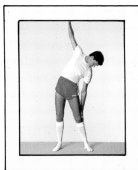
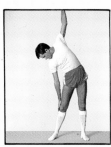

SKY REACHES

Stand erect and extend your right arm straight up while dropping your left arm down your outer thigh.
Repeat 10× on each side.

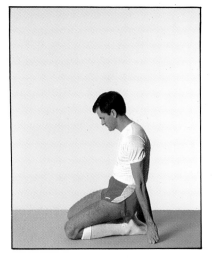

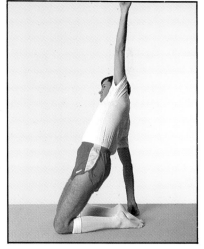

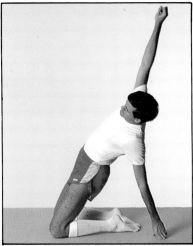

THE WONDER SPREAD

Kneel on the floor with your hips resting on your heels and your hands on the floor behind your feet.

Raise your buttocks up off your heels and as you are doing so, reach straight up with your left hand. Then move your left hand over to the right side of your body.

Return to starting position and repeat on the other side. Repeat 10×.

► *TUMMY FLATTENERS*

Once you're really into keeping fit and trim, you'll be looking for new routines to help fight the battle of the bulge. Let's really get cracking on flattening your stomach with these exercises.

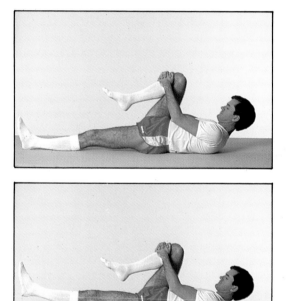

BELLY REPS

Lie on your back with both legs flat on the ground. Keep your left leg extended while you clasp the right knee with your hands.

Tuck your head near your chest as you slowly raise your left leg off the floor and try to sit up until your chin touches your right knee.

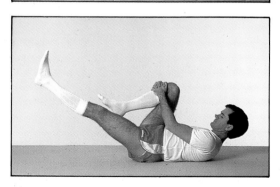

Return to starting position. Repeat, using the other knee. Do 20 repetitions (20×).

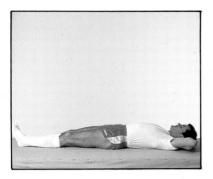

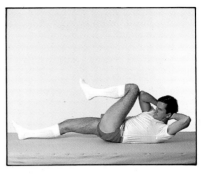

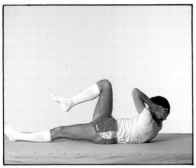

TUMMY TONER

Lie on back with your hands clasped behind head. Bend your right knee slightly.
Bring the left knee toward your head as you extend the right leg fully and touch the right elbow to the left knee.
Repeat with left elbow to right knee. Repeat 10×.

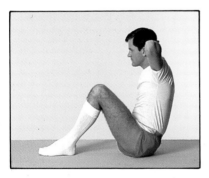

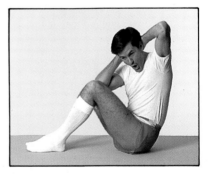

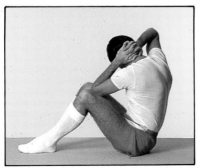

TWIST AND SHOUT

Sit on the floor with your hands clasped behind your head with your knees bent so that your feet are flat on the floor.
Twist your torso until your right elbow touches your left knee.
Return to starting position and repeat with left elbow to right knee. Repeat 15×.

▶ *PUSH-UPS*

Push-ups are an excellent way to develop the arm, shoulder, and chest muscles without resorting to heavy weight-training. The secret ·is repetitions. The more you can do, the stronger you'll become. Start out by finding your limit and then increasing it by one each day.

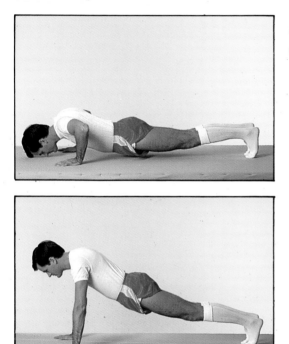

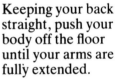

STANDARD PUSH-UPS

Lie on the floor face down with your legs together and hands under your shoulders.

Keeping your back straight, push your body off the floor until your arms are fully extended.

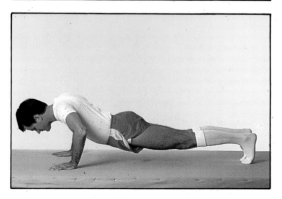

Then lower the body until your chin touches the floor. Do 10 repetitions (10×).

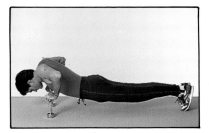

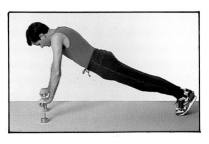

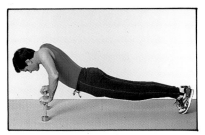

DIPS

Place hands on a solid support positioned under each shoulder. Keeping your back straight, push your body up until your arms are fully extended. Then lower the body so chin touches the floor. Repeat 5×.

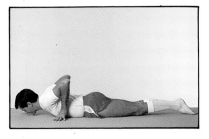

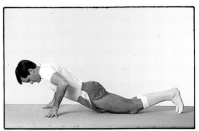

FINGER PUSH-UPS

Lie on the floor face down with your legs together and your fingers positioned on the floor under each shoulder.

Keeping your back straight, push your body off the floor using your toes and fingertips to support the weight.

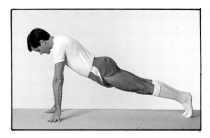

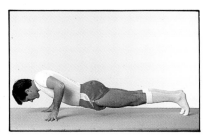

Continue upwards until your arms are fully extended.

Then lower the body until your chin touches the floor. Repeat 10×.

▶ PULL-UPS

Pull-ups are a great way to develop the arms, shoulders, upper back muscles, and even the abdominals. Ideally, they should be done from a bar that you can grasp with both hands. However, you can use a tree limb, a ceiling beam, or even the moldings on the top of doorways. Before jumping up and grabbing a makeshift bar, test it first to be sure it can support your weight. For greater abdominal workouts during the pull-ups, try tucking your knees up near your chest.

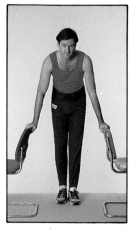

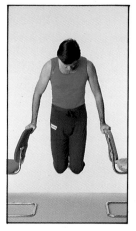

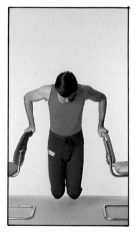

CHAIR-UPS

Place two chairs on either side of you with their backs facing your shoulders about 2 feet apart.

Grasp the top of the chairs and tuck up your knees so you're off the floor.

Dip down slowly until your shoulders are at the level of your hands.
Raise up to the starting position.
Repeat 10×.

STANDARD PULL-UPS

Grasp the bar with your palms facing you. Hang still for a second and then pull your body upward until your chin is level with the bar. Slowly drop down to the starting position. (Note: try not to "pump" your legs, as this will detract from the upper body workout. Do 10 repetitions (10×).

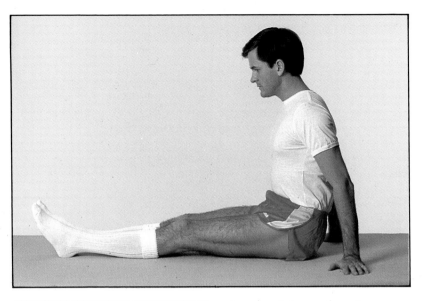

HIP-UPS

Sit on the floor with your legs fully extended together, in front of you and the palms of your hands flat on either side. Keep your back straight.

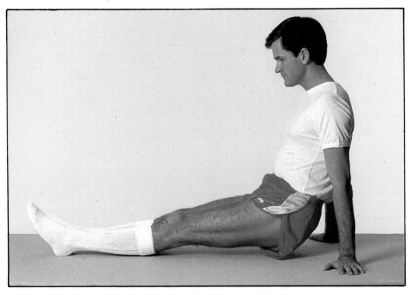

Press your body up until your buttocks are off the floor, still keeping your back as straight as possible. Hold for three seconds and then return to the starting position. Repeat 10×.

▶ *LEG DEVELOPERS*

When you can't get out and jog a few miles, you need some other exercise or your legs begin to lose their tone and development. For those of you who prefer to workout on your own, not wishing to join the sweating masses at the health club, here are a few home exercises guaranteed to put muscles on those legs.

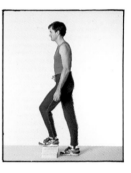

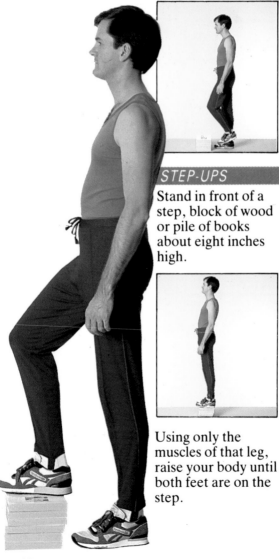

STEP-UPS

Stand in front of a step, block of wood or pile of books about eight inches high.

Place the left foot on the support.

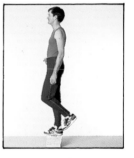

Using only the muscles of that leg, raise your body until both feet are on the step.

Step backward with left foot, bringing your body back to the starting position. Repeat, starting with the right foot. Repeat 10 times (10×) for each leg.

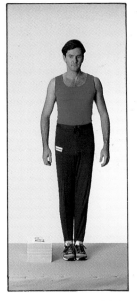
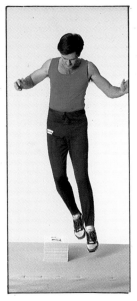
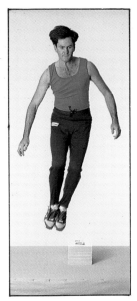

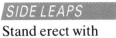
SIDE LEAPS

Stand erect with both feet together next to a pile of books at least 10 inches high.

Jump sideways over the pile, landing with both feet on the other side.

Then jump back to the starting position. Repeat 10×.

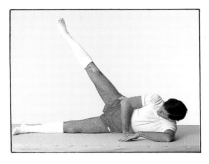
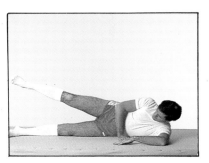

SIDE LEG RAISES

Lie on your left side on the floor with your legs extended, your weight supported by your arms.

Keeping the left leg on the floor, raise the other leg as high as possible.

Then lower the leg to the starting position. Repeat 15× on each side.

ARM PUNCHES

Sometimes you can combine two or three exercises and devise a new routine that benefits several different muscles. When you see a professional boxer throwing a punch, for example, watch how the real power begins in the fighter's stomach and back. A boxer's strength travels up his body, through his arms and finally explodes out of the fists. Before you go running off to challenge the heavyweight champion, try some of these exercises to strengthen your back, stomach, chest, and arms.

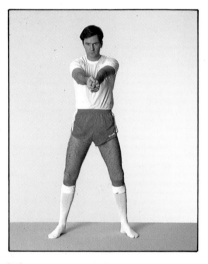

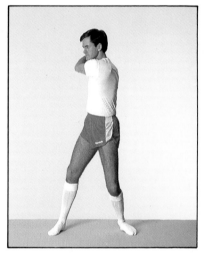

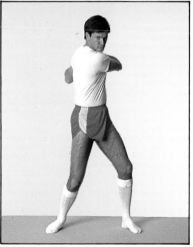

BASEBALL SWING

Stand erect with your legs apart and knees slightly bent and clasp your hands together with your arms straight ahead.

Then swing your arms to the right and round as far as you can and back.

Repeat the same exercise, swinging the other way. Do 10 repetitions (10×).

SWINGING ARMS

Stand erect with your legs apart and knees slightly bent, and raise your arms to either side.

Twist your body as you swing your arms so that your right hand faces in the direction as your toes and your left hand points away behind you.

Swing back the other way through the starting position. Repeat 20×.

▶ *CHEST REPS*

If you thought that only Tarzan and Superman had massive chests, wait until you try these exercises. You can expand and develop the arm and chest muscles at the same time, without the use of weights. Follow these directions and the chest is easy!

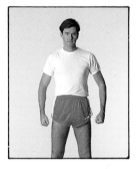

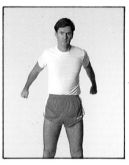

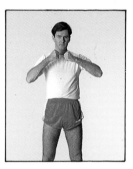

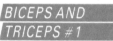
BICEPS AND TRICEPS #1

Stand erect with your feet apart and with your arms at your sides.

Then curl your arms up until the fists are almost at chin level.

Push arms back through the original position until fully extended behind you. Return to the original position. Repeat 20×.

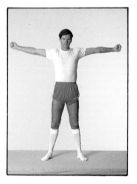

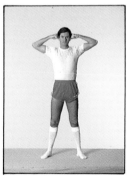

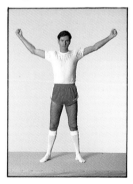

BICEPS AND TRICEPS #2

Stand erect with your feet apart and extend your arms to either side.

Flex your arms and bend them at the elbow until your fists rest on the sides of your head.

Push the arms, flexed, back to either side. Repeat 20×.

CHEST PULL

Stand erect with your feet apart.

Bend your arms, make fists and tuck your arms across the front of your chest.

Then bring your forearms out to the side.

Keep flexing and pulling the forearms back to the chest. Do 20 repetitions (20×)

▶ *JUMPING ROPE*

Some exercises are more fun than others. Every child in America has jumped rope for fun. Now's the time to start jumping rope for exercise and fitness. Rope work develops your strength, flexibility, and endurance. It's also a great way to work on the hand–eye coordination that you'll need in most sports.

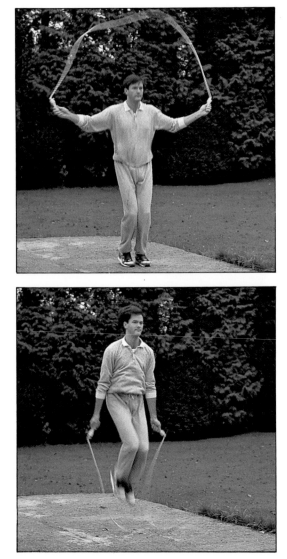

BASIC ROPE WORK

Stand erect with your feet together and the rope behind you, with your knees slightly bent. Bring the rope over the head and down in front of you.

As the rope nears your feet, jump, passing the rope under your feet. Bring the rope back behind you. Repeat 50 times (50×).

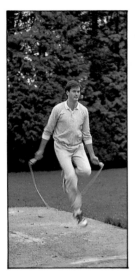 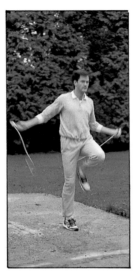 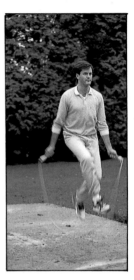

RUNNING ROPE WORK

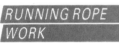

Stand erect with your feet together and swing the rope over your head and down in front of you.

As the rope nears your feet, leap over it with your right foot. Continue passing the rope, lifting the left leg. Keep swinging the rope.

During the next pass, leap over it with your left foot, then raise your right. (Note: if you do this fast enough, it'll feel as if you're jogging through the rope.) Repeat 50×.

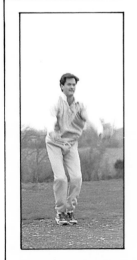 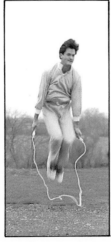

SHUFFLING ROPE WORK

Stand with your feet together and knees slightly bent.

Bring the rope around your body as in the basic rope work exercise but throw both legs from side to side as the rope passes beneath you. Repeat 50×.

▶ *JOGGING IN PLACE*

Even though it's a good fundamental exercise, jogging can get boring. Some of you have probably discovered that watching TV or listening to music while jogging helps the minutes fly by. Another way to break up the routine is by working out your upper body as you jog in place. Try some of these jogging add-ons and maybe you too will become hot to trot!

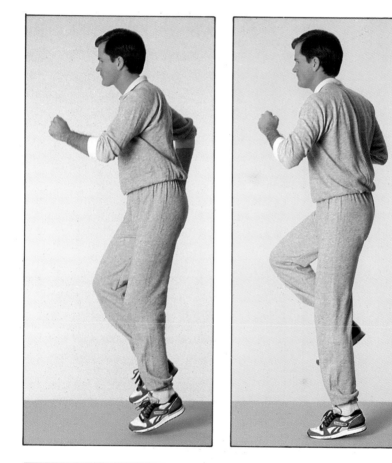

BASIC JOG

On a soft mat begin jogging in place. Remember to strike the floor with your toes first before rolling toward your heel.

As a variation on the basic jog, keep the knees lower but bring your heel up to your buttocks when the other leg is planted. Jog for 10 minutes.

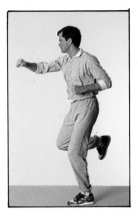 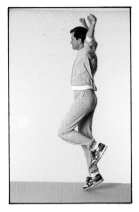 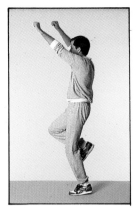

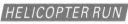

HIT AND RUN

Begin the basic jog until your body's warmed up. Throw punches with alternate hands as you jog. Try to put some force into each punch. Do 10 repetitions (10×) for each hand.

HELICOPTER RUN

Begin the basic jog and then extend your arms out to the side.

Circle your fists to either side as you continue running. Keep your stomach tight and try to pull your arms toward the walls. Continue for three minutes.

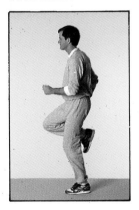 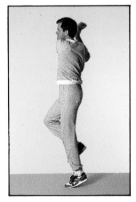 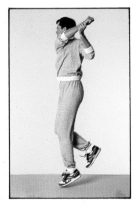

ARM-BUSTING RUN

Begin the basic jog, curl your arms and flex them.

As you run, alternate bringing one arm up past your chest to your chin with the other arm.

Repeat 20× for each arm.

▶ *JUMPING JACKS*

One of the first exercises you ever learned was probably jumping jacks. Easy to learn and good for fitness and coordination, jumping jacks should still be a part of your daily workout. Besides being a good change from jogging, jumping jacks help develop arm and shoulder strength.

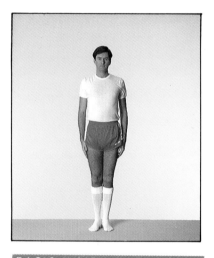

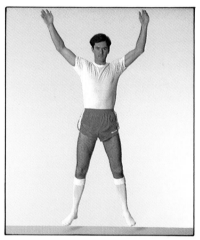

BASIC JUMPING JACK

Stand erect with your feet together.

Jump up as you throw your legs to either side, moving your arms outward from your sides until they meet over your head.

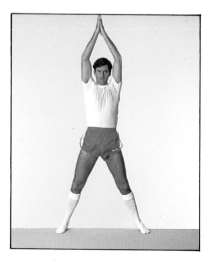

Time it so that your hands meet at the same time that your feet hit the floor. Then jump up and return to the starting position. Do 50 repetitions (50×).

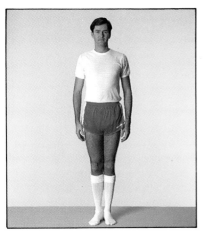

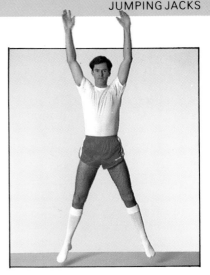

JUMPING JACK BE NIMBLE

Stand erect with your feet together.

Jump up as you throw your legs to either side, while bringing your hands outward from your sides to above your head.

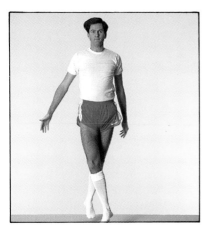

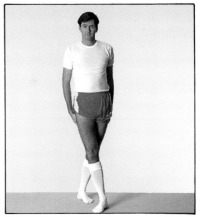

Then jump up again; as your hands return to your sides, bring your legs back down and cross them with the right foot in front of the left when they land.

Repeat the exercise alternating the landing so that one foot is always in front of the other. Repeat 25×.
Note: To increase your coordination and flexibility, start doing the basic jumping jacks and then double the tempo. Jump for two minutes at the higher speed.

►*A LOW-IMPACT AEROBIC WORKOUT*

The benefits of aerobic workouts include greater flexibility, endurance, and strength. Low-impact aerobics are special because they are designed to reduce the threat of injury to the lower body.

In the traditional high-impact program, both feet are simultaneously off the ground, and shin splints, twisted ankles, and foot and knee sprains can result. The theory behind the low-impact routine is that keeping one foot constantly on the mat places less stress on the legs. However, since the ultimate goal of any aerobic workout is to increase the heartbeat to a total of 175 percent of your normal pulse rate, you'd really have to shake, rattle, and roll if you couldn't jump off the mat with both feet. Low-impact aerobics therefore frequently require you to work with three- or five-pound weights in your hands. The added weight makes the upper body work harder and makes up for the lack of high impact by the feet on the mat.

To make it easier for you to learn our low-impact routine, we'll use some of the traditional exercises already explained. Use two easy-to-hold objects, weighing no more than five pounds each. Hold one in each hand and follow the program below. For example, if we're doing chest pulls, you'll be pulling those five-pound weights toward your chest. It won't be as easy as it seems, but the cardiovascular benefits will be very rewarding.

The trick to aerobics is to do the routine to thumping, rhythmic music. The music should supply the beat to keep you going through the routine. And speaking of routine, we won't tell you how many repetitions to do for each part of the workout. You should do it at your own pace. The rule of thumb, however, is that after you've finished the warm-ups, the actual aerobic portion of your workout should be at least 10 minutes for you to get any real heart and lung benefit.

Start your workout by doing the basic warm-up described earlier. Note: If you're susceptible to foot injuries, omit the jogging from the warm-up.

Do the following exercises while moving the legs up and down alternately. The secret of low-impact aerobics is to keep moving, as if you were doing dance steps. Keep a good beat to the music. Hold the weights in your hands and get into it. Since you really have to work at low-impact aerobics to get any benefit, the more you kick and drive the legs, the more you'll reap the aerobic rewards. Here's a suggested low-impact aerobic routine, based on the exercises described earlier. You can do them in any order that suits you. Remember, your low-impact routine must last at least 10 minutes.

- Side Bends while kicking legs, alternating each leg.
- Doorknob Turns, while raising alternating knees.
- Shoulder Shrugs, while raising alternating knees.
- Waist Leans, while kicking out alternating legs.
- The Punch, while kicking out alternating legs.
- Swinging Arms, while kicking out alternating legs.
- Chest Pulls, while raising alternating knees.
- Biceps and Triceps, while alternating knee raises.

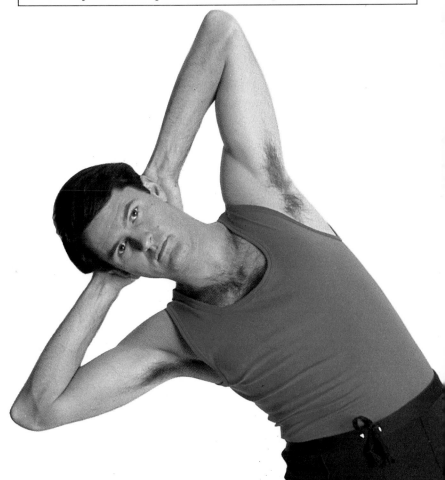

▶ PROS AND CONS OF LOW-IMPACT AEROBICS

Many people suffer leg injuries from traditional aerobic workouts, and some have turned to the new, low-impact exercises. Exercises such as simulated rope jumping or jumping jacks, so popular in regular aerobics, are missing from the low-impact regimen since one foot remains on the ground at all times.

Low impact doesn't mean low intensity. You still exercise at a fast pace to build up the cardiovascular system. To make up for the lack of jumping, some people hold or swing weights in their hands during the workout. Low-impact aerobics will improve your health and help keep lower-body injuries to a minimum.

The problem with low-impact aerobics is that, depending on the level of the program, you may not be pushing the heart hard enough to derive any aerobic benefits. The optimum pulse range to achieve in an aerobic workout is your normal pulse plus 75 percent. In other words, if your pulse is normally 100 beats per minute, your rate during aerobic exercise should be around 175. This rate may be impossible to achieve during a low-impact workout. In fact, if you're in good cardiovascular shape and then go on a low-impact program, you may be reducing your heart health, oxygen utilization, and energy reserve.

Another drawback of the low-impact system is that for many of the weight exercises you have to strain and stretch your muscles just to maintain your balance. Since your feet are usually on the floor, this can overwork the muscles of the upper body. Low-impact exercisers suffer from tendinitis and even bursitis of the shoulders and arms. Many low-impact exercises are done on the floor standing erect and there is also a tendency toward ankle injuries.

Perhaps the best solution is to alternate the routine. All beginners should start with a low-impact workout until their bodies become acclimated to aerobics. Once the muscles have been properly introduced to the wonders of aerobics, it's time for the high-impact workout to get the heart in shape.

Weights are commonly used in low-impact aerobic exercise programs.

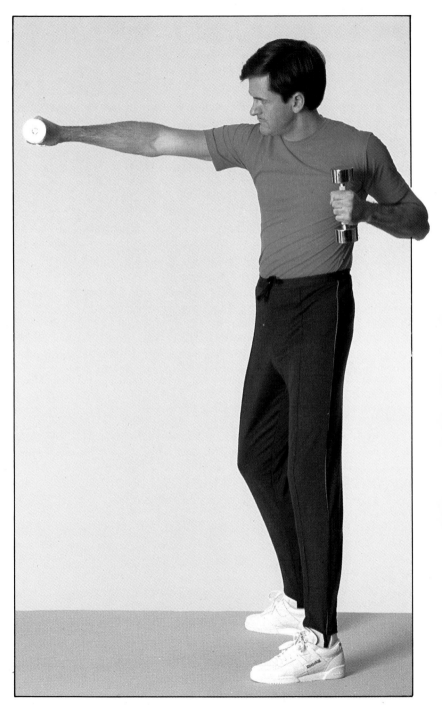

▶ A HIGH-IMPACT AEROBIC WORKOUT

The benefits of high-impact aerobics are that your body will feel stronger, more flexible, and more alive. Since your feet and legs will take a lot of pounding, get yourself a good pair of workout shoes, put on some thumping music to jump around to and go for it!

THE WARM-UP

Do the basic warm-up as detailed earlier. After you've done the basic exercises, it's time to start the aerobic warm-ups. Begin by clapping your hands as your step to the right and slide your left leg over to join the right. Repeat the motion to the left. Do that for about a minute. Breathe deeply, as this is going to be an aerobic workout and that means you'll be burning up oxygen.

Then begin a nice slow jog as you occasionally raise both your arms over your head. The pace should be moderate now as your body warms up. After jogging for a minute, do 10 jumping jacks, clapping your hands over the head.

THE AEROBICS

Now that you're all warmed up, it's time to boogie! The following exercises should be done at a rapid pace. With each one you'll want to be jogging, hopping, or doing jumping jacks to the music. Don't give up and stand still. If you feel tired, then just jog slowly in place until you catch your breath. If you begin to feel dizzy or feel a flutter in your heart — stop. You may want to consult a doctor before beginning any aerobic workout. Do these exercises in any order you want:

- Chest Pulls
- The Punch
- Trunk Turns
- Giant Arm Swings
- Waist Tilts
- Knee Grinds
- Biceps and Triceps #1
- Biceps and Triceps #2
- Simulated Rope Work (without the rope)
- Basic Jumping Jacks

Feel free to use any of the exercises in this book to assemble your own high-impact aerobic workout. Just remember the trick here is to keep those legs hopping, skipping, and jumping. Keep the aerobics going for at least 10 minutes, 15 if possible.

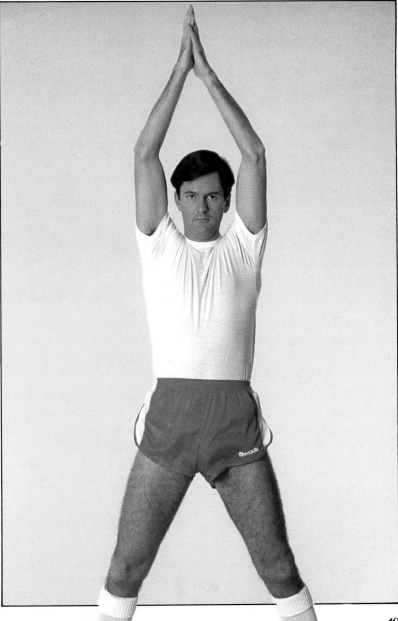

▶ *AEROBIC WORKOUT INJURIES*

You're 10 minutes into your aerobic workout. The sweat is pouring from your face. Your muscles are toned and you're finally in step with the rest of the class to the rhythm of the music. Suddenly, just as you begin to think that life can't get much better than this, you feel a jolt of pain race through your leg. Figuring it's only a spasm, you keep on jumping until the pain finally gets so intense, they have to carry you off the floor.

Congratulations. You've just joined the 50 percent club. Over 50 percent of those who participate in aerobics suffer some injury to their legs, back, and/or upper body. Most of the injuries are caused by the impact of your feet landing repeatedly on the matted floor. The feet absorb most of the stress, but some of it moves up the body, affecting the legs and back. The majority of upper-body aerobic injuries occur during low-impact workouts.

In high-impact aerobics, where both your feet spend time off the ground simultaneously, most injuries are to the shins. The injuries, ranging from simple inflammation to tearing of the membrane between the tibia and fibula, are caused by the compression of your body as you land, putting stress on the lower leg. To prevent the common ailment of shin splints:

Do a series of warm-ups before the aerobics.

Make sure your shoes have ample shock absorbers in the midsole and inner sole.

If you have shin splints, ice down the leg area after your workout to reduce the inflammation. A sign that you may be developing shin splints is when the lower leg feels very tight after a workout. If that's the case, try warming up longer and exercising on a softer surface.

High-impact workouts can also cause tendinitis, which is an inflammation of a tendon. This occurs when a tendon is overused and shortened, most often caused by landing on your toes too much. To prevent tendinitis, stretch the tendons of the leg by keeping your heels on the floor as you lean forward against a wall. A sign that you already have tendinitis is swelling and pain when you move the affected joint. If tendinitis develops try to rest the leg, apply ice and elevate.

If aerobics cause you back pain, then you should try to strengthen the abdominal muscles with sit-ups. The abdominals help take the pressure off the back.

Low-impact workouts tend to injure the upper body because of the common practice of swinging weights to compensate for the lack of jumping movement. The most common injuries are tendinitis in the arms, pulled backs, and strains. If you suffer an injury, stop your activity and apply ice if possible. As with any injury, if the pain persists, see a doctor.

COMMON LEG INJURIES

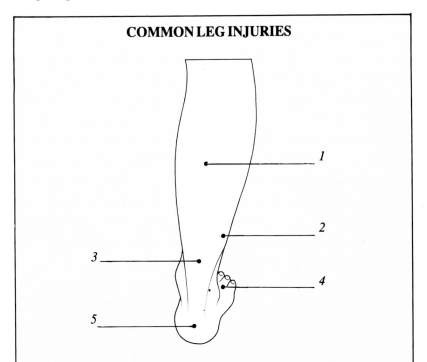

Aerobic injuries include:
1 shin splints caused by stress on the lower leg and calf strain caused by overuse of the calf muscle.
2 outer shin muscle strain or peroneal tendon strain caused by working out on an uneven surface or in such a way that the body weight falls too much on the outside of the foot
3 Achilles tendon damage caused by overuse and too much running on the toes or poorly fitting workout shoes
4 March fractures (stress fractures) in the small bones of the foot following excessive roadrunning
5 heelbone lumps (bursae) caused by shoe friction

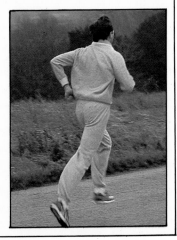

▶ *WARMING DOWN*

Too many exercisers who are doing workouts for the first time are so happy when they've finished the strenuous part of the workout that they race off for the showers. Soon their muscles may begin to cramp and spasm and they limp their way to the corner drugstore for liniment and rubbing alcohol.

After every exercise session or sports competition, you have to warm your body down. The rule of thumb calls for you to spend as much time warming down as you did warming up! All those muscles that have now been exercised need time to readjust to their normal status. Otherwise, they may tear or pull even though no further stress is placed on them.

If you've completed a fast-paced aerobic workout, your system needs time to slow down. Going from aerobics directly to a hot shower, without a slow warming down, may cause the cardiovascular system to go into shock. Don't forget, you've just gotten your heart pumping at a rate 75 percent more than it's accustomed to! After an aerobic workout, spend a few minutes doing the same type of exercises you did during the aerobic warm-up. For example, try shuffling back and forth as you clap your hands.

If you've incorporated some abdominal exercises, you should take the time to do some simple stretches. Remember, most abdominal exercises and aerobics place a strain on the back. All that tightening and jumping may compress some of the vertebrae in the spine. Let's elongate the spine and warm down properly:

- Lie on your back with your hands clasped around your knees. Gently pull your knees onto your chest and hold for 5 seconds.
- Release your knees and let them both fall to the left side. Relax your body, letting the weight of the legs do the work.
- Gently move your knees to the right side and relax.
- Kneel on all fours and arch your back. Slowly push yourself forward, sliding your hands until your stomach rests on the ground and your arms are directly in front of you. Hold for 5 seconds. Then pull up to the starting position.
- Stand erect and do Deep Breaths.
- Now it's time for your reward . . . hit the showers!

Complete your warming down by *breathing deeply while standing erect.*

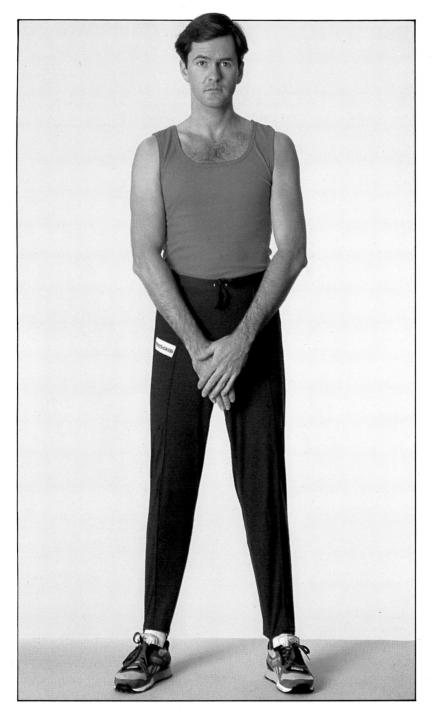

▶ *WEIGHT TRAINING*

Weight training is a way to develop muscle strength in specific parts of the body. Through proper methods you can isolate muscle groups to get the maximum benefit from the exercises. Of course, any health club has ample weight-training facilities, including dumbbells, barbells, and some of the more sophisticated machines that incorporate set weights in easy-to-use stations.

For our purposes, we'll concentrate on a few exercises that you can do at home with a simple set of dumbbells and a barbell. Remember to warm up first before you hit those weights. If you find that an exercise is getting too easy to do, don't do more repetitions — use heavier weights instead.

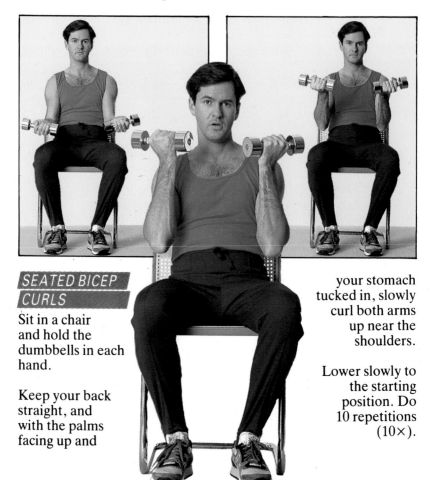

SEATED BICEP CURLS

Sit in a chair and hold the dumbbells in each hand.

Keep your back straight, and with the palms facing up and your stomach tucked in, slowly curl both arms up near the shoulders.

Lower slowly to the starting position. Do 10 repetitions (10×).

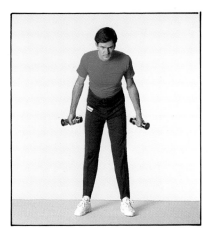

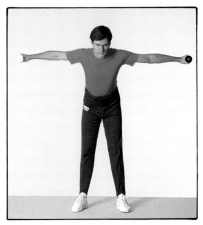

DUMBBELL ARM SWINGS

Grasp the dumbbells with your palms facing your sides and lean over from the waist, keeping your back straight.

Slowly, raise the dumbbells out to the sides until your arms are parallel to the floor. Return to starting position. Repeat 10×.

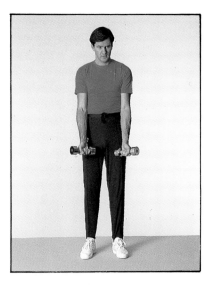

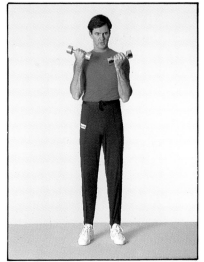

DUMBBELL CURLS

Stand erect with your legs close together, holding the dumbbells, palms up, down around your upper thighs.

Keep your upper body motionless and pull the dumbbells up, using your forearms, to your shoulders. Return to starting position. Repeat 10×.

TRICEP PRESSES

Sit or stand with your back straight, take one dumbbell and hold it directly over one shoulder, arm extended.

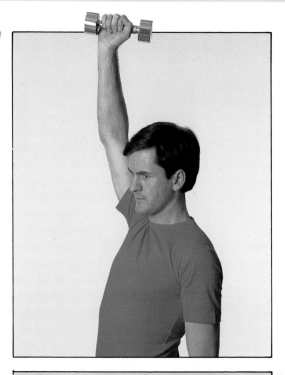

Use your free arm to brace the other's bicep by grasping it between the elbow and the shoulder.

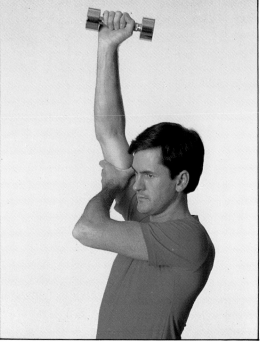

Then slowly lower
the dumbbell behind
you until it almost
touches your upper
back.

Slowly raise the
dumbbell to the
starting position.
Repeat 5×.

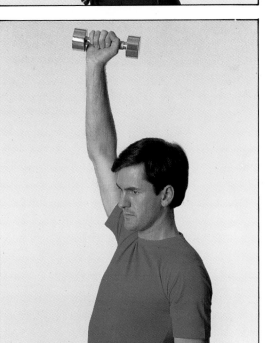

▶ *PREVENTING BAD BACKS*

Almost any type of physical exertion is capable of hurting your back. You can hurt your back doing anything from carrying out the trash to mowing the lawn. So if you're planning to exercise to keep fit, you want to take special precautions to keep your back from being injured.

The best way to help prevent back injuries is to warm up before working out. The more limber and flexible the muscles surrounding the back are, the less likely it is that they'll pull or tear. Select some of the traditional warm-ups and get into the habit of doing them before exercise or playing sports.

Some athletes are puzzled that simple jogging can injure the back. The constant pounding that your legs take when you jog is not completely absorbed by your lower body. Some of the vibrations carry on through the pelvic region, eventually settling on the spinal column. If you have back pain from jogging, try purchasing a pair of running shoes with more cushioning in the midsole and inner sole. You should also look into running on softer surfaces. Clay is always preferable to concrete!

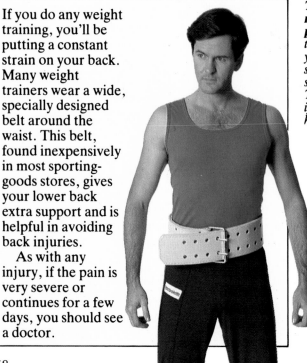

If you do any weight training, you'll be putting a constant strain on your back. Many weight trainers wear a wide, specially designed belt around the waist. This belt, found inexpensively in most sporting-goods stores, gives your lower back extra support and is helpful in avoiding back injuries.

As with any injury, if the pain is very severe or continues for a few days, you should see a doctor.

Try and maintain good posture at all times, keeping your back straight and your shoulders back. Take special care if you are lifting heavy weights.

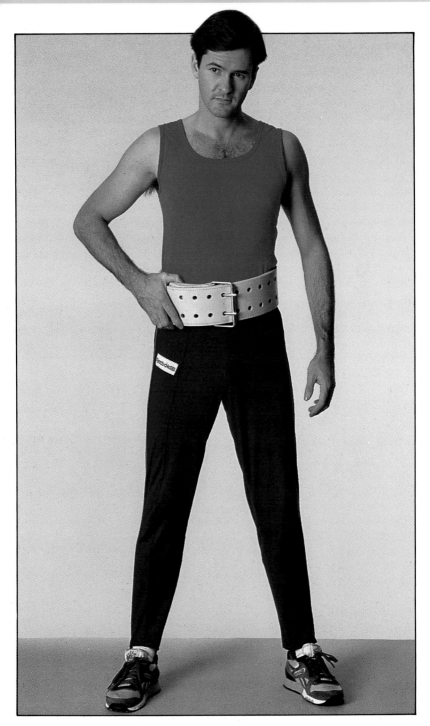

▶ *PROPER FOOTWEAR*

The most important piece of equipment you can own is a good pair of work-out shoes. Every time you jog or participate in an aerobic workout, you are transferring 3 times your body weight to the delicate bones and tissues of the feet. For the average weekend jogger, this amounts to over 100 tons of force applied to your feet for every mile. If you're going to continue putting your best foot forward, you must have the proper footwear.

Before you go running out to the store, sit down and take a good look at your feet. The type of work-out shoe you'll need is dictated by the shape and structure of your feet. You'll have to determine whether your feet pronate, supinate, or are neutral. A simple test is to walk across a dry floor with damp feet and then examine the footprints. If your feet pronate (also known as being flat-footed), each puddle/footprint will look like an outline of the entire foot. If so, you'll need shoes that provide more support. Look for a wide sole and a thick, hard upper. Don't go for heavy padding, since this might just exaggerate your problem. Instead, get shoes with hard midsoles and inner soles.

If each footprint on the floor just shows the toes and the ball of the foot, then you are a supinator, a person with a high arch. If you supinate, buy work-out shoes with cushioned outer, inner and mid-soles for better shock absorption.

If your footprint shows the toes, ball, and edges of the foot, you

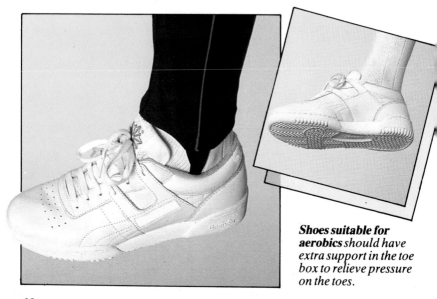

Shoes suitable for aerobics should have extra support in the toe box to relieve pressure on the toes.

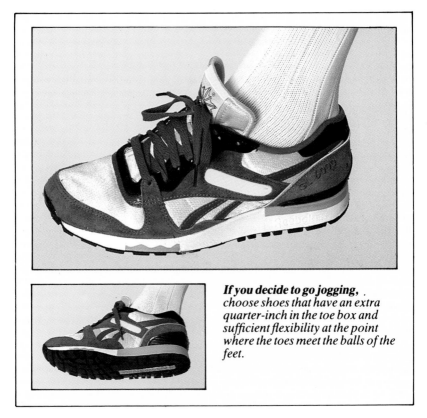

If you decide to go jogging, choose shoes that have an extra quarter-inch in the toe box and sufficient flexibility at the point where the toes meet the balls of the feet.

are blessed with neutrality. Purchase work-out shoes that provide cushioned shock-absorption and support.

After you've determined your foot type, it's time to buy the work-out shoes. Now you have to make a distinction. Are you a jogger or are you purchasing shoes for aerobics? What's the difference? If you are a jogger, you are constantly striding forward with your heel striking first and then rolling toward the toes. Select a shoe that gives you about an extra quarter-inch in the toe box. Make sure that the shoe has enough flexibility at the point where the balls of your feet meet the toes, so that the shoe will bend when you do!

If you're buying shoes for aerobics, remember that in most work-outs your toes strike the ground first and then you press down, using the heel to help absorb the shock. Make sure your aerobics shoe has extra support in the toe box to help relieve the pounding on the delicate toes. The importance of buying the correct footwear cannot be stressed enough: most jogging and aerobic injuries are preventable, as long as the proper shoes are worn.

▶ *PROPER CLOTHING*

The clothing you select for your workout helps determine how healthy your exercise will be. Wearing the proper clothes allows your body to breathe, to perspire, and to maintain enough heat to prevent muscle spasms and cramps.

For most indoor and outdoor warm-weather workouts it's generally enough to wear a pair of socks, an athletic supporter, a pair of shorts, and a T-shirt. Since you're exercising in a warm environment, you should wear clothes that allow your body to breathe and perspire. For this reason, try to stick with cotton-based clothing. Cotton is lightweight and porous, allowing for ventilation.

Too often the socks go neglected. We reach into the drawer, select any old pair of white athletic socks, and pull them on the feet. Paying attention to your footwear can save you from injuries down the road. Socks act as shock absorbers, so buy a pair that has cushioned heels and toes. The material of the sock is not that important, although cotton is lighter and more absorbant of perspiration than some of the polyester blends.

If you are working out outdoors in cold weather, you must wear heavier clothing. What you wear outside largely depends on how much you are willing to spend. Outdoor jogging suits, for example, can range from very inexpensive to a few hundred dollars for some of the new, scientifically tested models. The more expensive types will be lightweight and keep your body warm and toasty, and provide a barrier from the rain.

Don't let being on a tighter budget prevent you from working out outdoors. Remember that the more layers you put between you and Old Man Winter, the warmer you'll stay. A pair of sweat pants and a sweat shirt, over layers of long underwear, for example, will probably keep you warm. The problem with the sweats, of course, is that once they absorb your perspiration they can get very heavy.

Don't forget your head and hands. In cold weather wear a woolen cap to prevent any of your body heat from venting through your system's natural chimney, the head. Wear a pair of warm gloves to prevent chapping and heat escaping from the hands.

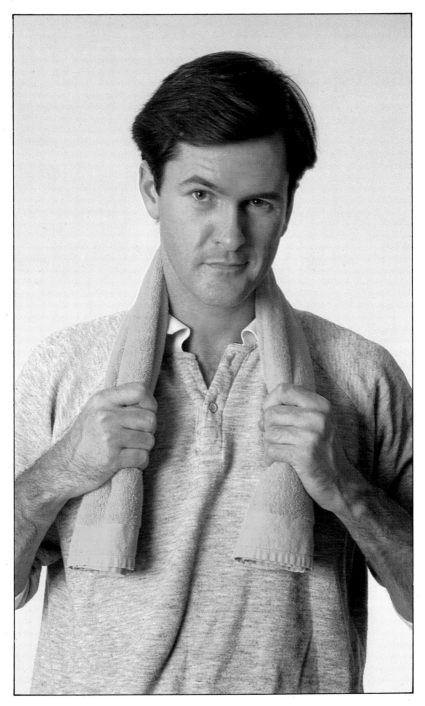

► *WATER EXERCISES*

Water provides an excellent source of resistance that makes even simple exercises fun and beneficial. Water exercises are often recommended for those with joint problems from injuries or from arthritis and bursitis.

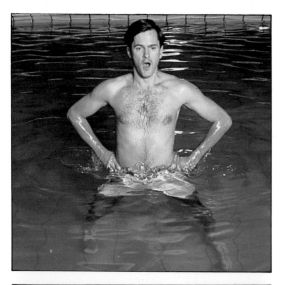

STANDING WATER #1

Stand with your feet slightly apart in waist- or chest-deep water and place hands on waist.

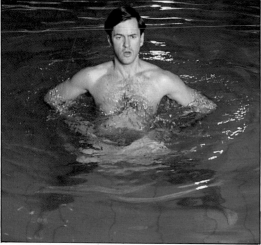

Jump up and extend legs sideward. Then jump up again and return legs to starting position. Do 10 repetitions (10×).

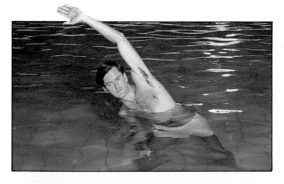

STANDING WATER #2

Stand in chest-deep water. Raise left arm straight up over head. Slowly stretch, bending to the right. Return to starting position. Alternate arms and bend over to the other side. Repeat 10×.

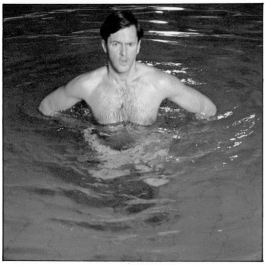

STANDING WATER #3

Stand in waist- or chest-deep water with hands on hips and feet together.

Lunge forward with one leg. At the same time, move the other leg back. Jump up and return to starting position. Alternate legs. Repeat 10×.

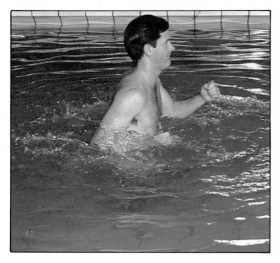

STANDING WATER #4

Stand in waist- or chest-deep water. With arms bent in running position, jog in place for 3 minutes.

POOL-SIDE DRILLS

By holding or leaning onto the side of the pool, you can isolate certain muscles during your workout.

POOL-SIDE #1

Stand at side of pool with back against wall and arms at sides. Raise left knee to chest and then extend left leg straight out. Drop leg to starting position. Alternate 5 times (5×).

POOL-SIDE #2

Stand at side of pool with back against wall. Raise left leg and clasp the calf with both arms, pulling it to the chest. Release leg and return to starting position. Alternate 5×.

POOL-SIDE #3

Hold onto side of pool with both arms, back toward wall. Let both legs float free. Bring both knees to chest. Release back to starting position. Repeat 10×.

POOL-SIDE #4

Hold onto side of pool with both arms, back toward wall. Let both legs float free. Swing legs far apart. Bring legs together, crossing left leg over right. Swing legs far apart. Bring legs together, crossing right leg over left. Repeat 10×.

POOL-SIDE #5

Stand at side of pool with back against wall. Hold onto wall with both hands. Lift left knee and move it to right. Return to standing position. Repeat with right knee. Alternate 5×.

CHEST PULLS IN WATER

The resistance provided by water can also be used to develop the upper body.

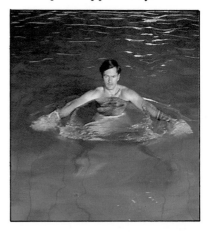

CHEST PULL #1

Stand in chest-high water with your arms extended in front under water and push them out to either side.

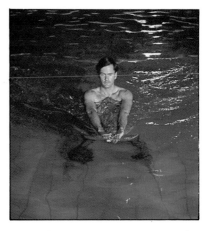

With open palms, drive the arms together until they meet in front. Do 10 repetitions (10×).

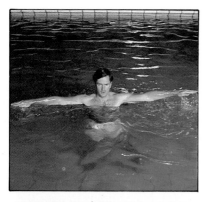

CHEST PULL #2

Stand in chest-high water. Extend arms to either side on top of water, palms down and open.
Drive the arms under water until they rest at sides. Pull arms back to surface of water. Repeat 10×.

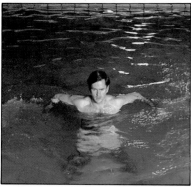

CHEST PULL #3

Stand in chest-high water away from the wall. Extend arms to either side on top of water, palms open. Push arms under the water toward the back until palms almost touch behind back. Pull arms forward to starting position. Repeat 5×.

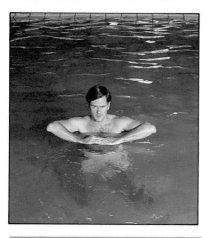

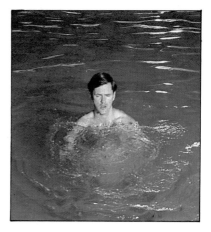

CHEST PULL #4

Stand in chest-high water. With arms bent in front and palms at chest, raise elbows.

Press the arms down toward the abdomen level. Pull arms back to starting position. Repeat vigorously 10×.

▶ VOLLEYBALL

Every beach in the country seems to come complete with sand, surf, bathing beauties, and a volleyball net. This energetic game requires the quickness and accuracy of the best of basketball and tennis. When you're fit and in shape, nothing can really compare with the thrill of jumping up in the air and coordinating your arms, hands, and upper body to deliver a game-winning spike.

Since volleyball requires the ability to jump, stretch, bend, and drive the ball, obviously you'll need to exercise to be in shape for the game.

One way to get the proper exercise for volleyball is to play some basketball, tennis, and squash. You'll be working out the same muscles you'll need for volleyball and having a good time to boot. And speaking of "booting," soccer is another good way to get in shape for volleyball. The constant running and last-second turns needed to play soccer are just right for the volleyball court!

During the off-season there are a number of simple exercises that prepare your muscles for volleyball. Side bends, trunk turns, and

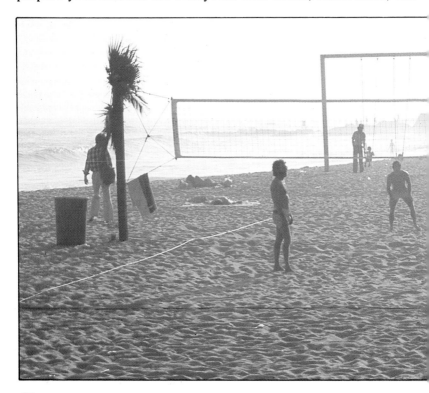

toe touches will strengthen the middle-torso muscles, enabling you to make those sharp turns. Since the abdomen plays such a big role in spiking the ball (it helps to generate power), do some crunches and some cycleless "bicycling."

Of course, you're also going to need powerful upper body and arm muscles. Do some chest pulls, push-ups, pull-ups, and biceps and triceps exercises.

If you're going to excel at volleyball, you'd better work on those upper and lower leg muscles. Do some knee clasps, lunges, and half-squats to get those legs in shape. Jumping rope, jogging, and high-impact aerobics will also prepare you for the game.

Before the game, take the time to jog around the court to get the circulation in your legs pumping. It's also a good idea to do some stretches. When your team is assembled, practice serving and spiking to get those specific muscles primed. Then go out there and enjoy the game. Remember . . . volleyball is the spike of life!

Volleyball *is a thrilling game requiring stamina and real all-round* *fitness. Warm up well before the game starts or you will pull a muscle.*

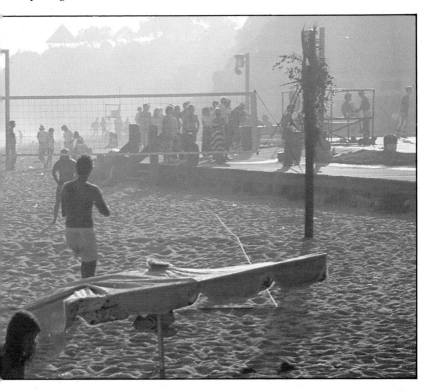

▶ *SKIING*

What an exhilarating feeling it is to fly down the side of a snow-covered mountain. It's even more exhilarating when you make it down with all your body parts intact. One way to enjoy the sport safely is to be in good skiing shape.

Skiing is a very strenuous activity. Using almost every muscle in your body, you coordinate your actions to react to the bumps and ridges as you attack the mountain. Flexibility, strength, and stamina are required to enjoy the day.

During the off-season, participate in any aerobic sport, including squash and soccer. Of course, high-impact aerobics is excellent for its endurance benefits and also as a way to develop crucial leg muscles.

Specific skiing exercises should include side bends, toe touches, head rolls, and giant arm circles to strengthen the muscles. Since the groin and thigh take such a pounding, it's also a great idea to give those a workout. Lunges, half-squats, and hurdle stretches all give much needed flexibility.

To get that upper torso in shape do pull-ups, push-ups, and some weight training. You must also fully develop your abdominal muscles to help you navigate down those trails. Crunches, knee clasps, and wonder spreads will keep that stomach nice and tight. Remember, you want to be in shape to tackle the mountain and you want to look your best in those tight-fitting ski outfits!

Jogging, jumping rope, and aerobics will help build up cardio-vascular strength. As the ski season approaches you may want to increase the time devoted to these exercises.

When you're on the top of the mountain, it's time for some preliminary warm-ups. Don't just buckle on those skis and take-off. You want to enjoy the whole day, don't you?

Loosen up those thighs with a few half-squats. Get those leg tendons in line with a few calf stretches. Do some chest pulls to wake up the upper torso. Head rolls and shoulder shrugs will make everything just about right. Then take a few deep breathes, pull on those goggles, and hit the snow!

Being in good skiing shape is essential to enjoying your skiing. Develop a high-impact aerobics program to build up your endurance and concentrate on exercises to build up general flexibility.

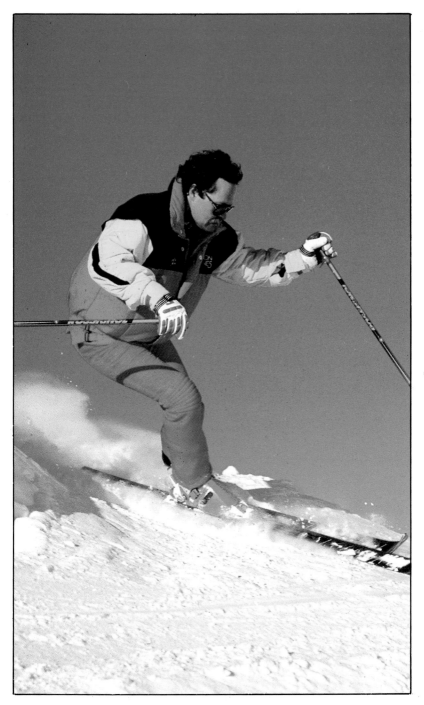

▶ *TENNIS*

Whether you're a touring professional or just like to bang the ball around on weekends, getting your body fit for tennis will improve your game and prevent injuries. Tennis requires muscle coordination and strength combined with stamina and you need to be very fit.

You work out a few days a week at the gym. Four days a week you do a few laps around the park. Then the weekend comes and it's time for tennis. On the court you volley for a few minutes and then, itching to blow away your opponent, you start the game. Two serves into the match and you get a cramp in your leg. Puzzled, you limp off the court, wondering what happened to all your physical preparation. What happened was that you may have been in great overall condition, but you didn't take the time to warm up adequately before the match.

To warm up properly you have to prepare the muscles for the exertion and the constant starting and stopping required in tennis.

A good tennis warm-up should include:

1. Jogging in place for a few minutes. This not only gets the heart pumping, but loosens up the leg muscles.
2. Stretching the legs. Pay special attention to the tendons in the leg by leaning against a wall with your heels on the ground.
3. Keeping the cover on the racquet, practice your forehand and backhand shots without hitting the ball. The cover provides greater resistance and builds arm strength.
4. Take the cover off and bounce a ball on alternate sides of the racquet to warm up the wrists and hands.
5. About ten minutes before the match, you and your opponent should hit the ball back and forth across the net. Although this should be done at a slow pace, it'll prepare the body for the more rigorous game.

During the week in your general exercise routine there are a few workouts that are especially good for tennis players. Include side bends, shoulder shrugs, trunk twists, push-ups, sit-ups, and some jogging and rope work.

Since gripping the tennis racquet requires strong hand muscles, try squeezing a tennis ball every so often. Squeeze and release, repeating this 20 times. Soon you'll be smashing those serves and lofting those lobs as if you were born with a racquet in your hand!

The game of tennis demands both stamina and short bursts of hard physical exertion. Follow a fitness routine to strengthen your back and torso muscles, your legs and your arms and hands.

▶ *GOLF*

Grabbing the clubs out of the trunk of the car, you race to the first tee, anticipating an afternoon of well-hit golf balls driving down the middle of the fairway. After sitting behind a desk all week you've really come to appreciate this weekend game in the country. Ball teed up, you take one or two practice swings and then step up to smack the ball. Soon you're skulking off into the woods attempting to find your golf ball. Miraculously, you find it wedged under an old, discarded radial tire. You bend over to pick it up and an excruciating pain attacks your back. You've just learned that although golf is a slow-paced game, it requires strength and stamina.

Your workouts during the week should include jogging and aerobics to increase your stamina. Even if you ride around in a golf cart, you'll need endurance to maintain your alertness during the four hours on the course. To develop your strength to enable you to hit the ball farther, try lifting some light weights on the non-aerobic days. Also do some push-ups, sit-ups, and trunk twists. To strengthen your hands to grip the club, you can repeatedly squeeze a tennis ball or even make a fist.

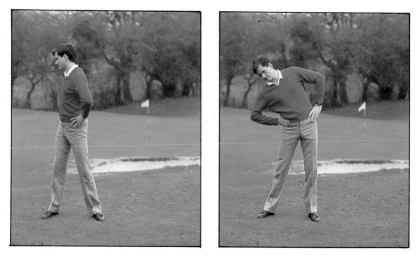

Take the time to limber up *before teeing off.*

When you arrive at the golf course, take a few minutes to limber up as soon as you get out of the car. Surprisingly, some golfers hurt their backs by jumping out of the car and bending over to get their clubs! Do some slow side bends and trunk twists to get the back nice and limber. Then check in, and go to the first tee.

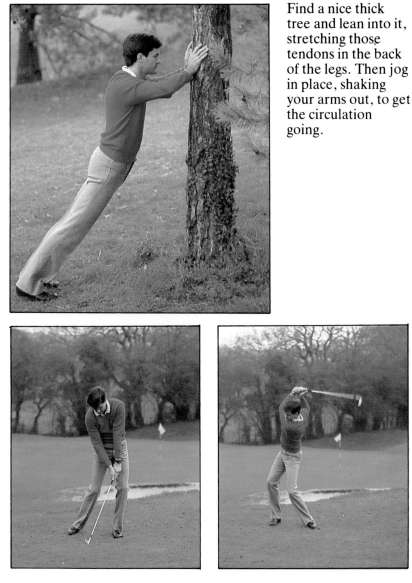

Find a nice thick tree and lean into it, stretching those tendons in the back of the legs. Then jog in place, shaking your arms out, to get the circulation going.

Build up to the full swing of the club in stages.

Now it's time to grab a club. But leave your driver in the bag! Start out by swinging a nine iron, nice and easy. Take a few swings and then pull out a five iron, then a three iron, and finally the driver. In this way, you'll build up to swinging the heavier clubs. Then, once you've warmed up, get out there and break a hundred!

▶ *BICYCLING*

Remember when you were young and the first thing you did after school was race home, grab your bicycle, and zoom off into the neighborhood? You were able to live at that frenetic pace because young boys have flexible, supple muscles. Older guys have to exercise to keep that flexibility!

If you're just in average shape and attempt to race home after work and jump on your bicycle, you'll develop charley horses and cramps all over your body. Bicycling is vigorous exercise and although it's a great stamina-builder, you have to be in relatively good shape to begin with.

Since bicycling requires endurance and strongly developed legs, these are the areas that should be stressed in your daily workouts. Concentrate on trunk twists, side bends, push-ups, and sit-ups. A great exercise is copied directly from the motion required to pedal a bicycle. Lie on your back and place your hands against the base of the spine. Keeping your legs up in the air, and supporting your body with your hands, slowly carry out a pedaling motion. Start doing this for about three minutes at first, gradually increasing to ten.

Since you must have powerful legs to bicycle, spend some time working on the lower body. Do some leg raises while sitting in a chair. Go over to a staircase and do about 20 step-ups. They not only increase the muscle strength in your legs but also add to your stamina.

Once you're in bicycling shape, you still should spend some time warming up before jumping on the bicycle. Spread your legs wide apart, bend over to one side and grasp an ankle. Hold for a few seconds, and then repeat with the other ankle. Stretch out those tendons in the leg by leaning against a wall or tree, keeping those heels on the ground.

Since it's a good idea to start the heart pumping faster, jog in place for a minute or two. You can even try jogging while hunching forward slightly, copying the position on a bicycle.

Keep in shape, warm up before starting, and you'll have an enjoyable ride!

Bicycling, whether for pleasure or to and from the office, is great exercise. Warm up before you start, get in shape, and you'll cover the distance painlessly.

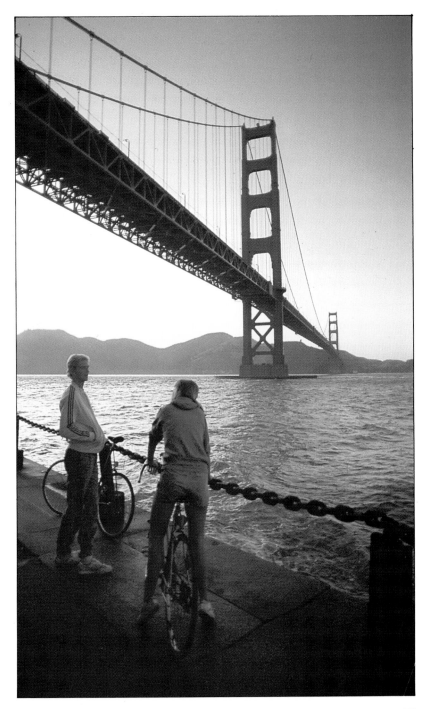

▶ *SOFTBALL*

All over the country, men are joining softball leagues and spending their early summer evenings and weekend mornings playing ball. Unfortunately, some of these guys spend their late evenings or weekend afternoons nursing pulled muscles and strained ligaments. Softball, like tennis and basketball, requires a variety of physical attributes. Since you have to run, throw, catch, and hit the elusive ball your body has to be in good overall condition. You need strong legs to run and a powerful upper body to drive one over the wall. Limber muscles come in handy for stretching to make those game-saving grabs.

During the off-season or any time between games, the softball player has to keep in shape. Aerobics and jogging are good conditioners for developing endurance. Jumping rope is another stamina-builder that also helps work on the upper body.

To build up and maintain strength you should work at exercises like trunk twists, side bends, and the usual assortment of push-ups and sit-ups. But if you really want to be the big hitter of the team,

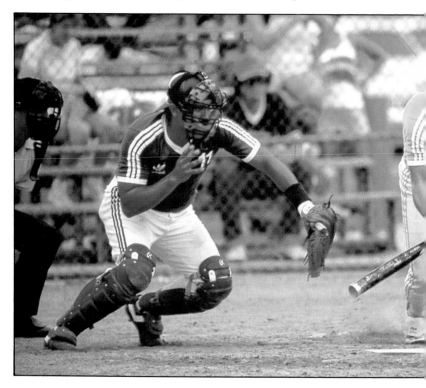

let's try to zap up those arm and chest muscles while still retaining flexibility. A good rule to remember is that after every strenuous muscle-building workout, take time to stretch out those limbs to keep them supple. Those weightlifters you see strutting around the gym could never have the bat speed needed to belt the softball. If you work out with free weights, for example, make sure to spend time warming down that specific muscle group. If you did a nice series of curls, building up those arms and chest, put the weights down, stretch out the arms, and slowly bring them back until they are extended behind your back. Hold for a few seconds. What you are doing is preventing those biceps from becoming muscle-bound!

Before the game you should spend half an hour getting warmed up and loose. Jog around the outfield and catch a few pop-ups. Then take a bat and slowly swing it back and forth to get the muscles limber. Once you begin to feel warmed up, take two bats and repeat the swinging. This will help you at bat, since you'll be able to swing one bat faster than the two. It's also a good idea to stretch out the legs. And keep active even after the game begins. Sitting around the dugout just gives your muscles time to tighten up.

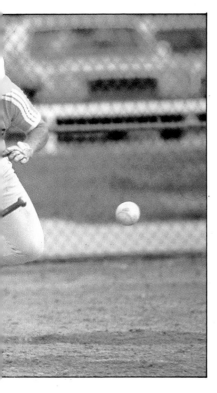

Running, throwing, hitting and catching the ball is hard work if you're not in shape. Work out to build up good overall fitness and try a little weight-training.

► *BASKETBALL*

If you've ever watched a professional basketball game you know how physical and draining the game can be. Running, leaping, passing, and shooting require responsive muscles and limitless endurance. For those of us who just play occasionally, the idea is to have fun and not get hurt.

To play basketball on any level, you have to condition your body by working out. Since so much of the game depends on leg strength, it's a good idea to concentrate on the lower body. Your upperbody strength will come from weights and isometrics. Remember, the more you can drive your arms upward, the higher you'll jump. Besides arm strength, you should work on flexibility through aerobics and stretching.

Since the legs are so vital, concentrate on building them up. Use repeated lunges to build up the thighs — it's the thighs that drive you upward, propelling you to the hoop. Another good thigh exercise calls for you to stand with your back against the wall. Slowly bring your leg up and clasp it with your hands, tuck your knee close to your chest and release. Then repeat with the other leg. The more powerful you make your thighs, the higher you'll be able to leap.

To develop leg quickness, try doing some step-ups on a staircase. If you can get to a long series of steps, such as those at an outdoor arena, work on those legs by running up to the top. Start slowly at first and after a few weeks it'll come easier.

Since the hands also play an important part in dribbling and passing, let's work on them too! Shake and twist your wrists, making them flexible and allowing you to snap those passes to your teammates!

A basketball game always has a lot of pushing under the basket, so you'll want to develop strong shoulders to keep your space and get that rebound. Push-ups and giant arm circles will strengthen the shoulders. Weight-training, of course, will also result in powerful shoulders and arms.

Before the game you should stretch out your muscles and jog around the court to get the circulation going. Your team should also go through lay-up and passing drills, all helping to get you accustomed to the court and also to limber up the basketball muscles.

Grab that rebound under the basket first every time and you'll win – basketball is a game of endurance. Get into shape with leg exercises, weight-training and isometrics.

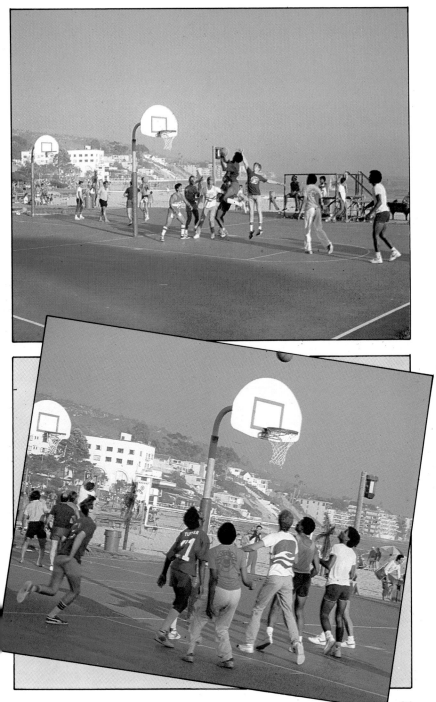

▶ *SWIMMING*

Swimming is a popular recreation that doesn't require you to spend hours in weight-training to enjoy it. However, you have to have limber, flexible muscles if you're going to swim for any length of time and not be stiff afterward.

One facet of your health that must be enhanced to enjoy swimming is your endurance and general cardiovascular fitness. In general, you can increase your stamina through aerobic workouts and jogging. The harder your work out, the stronger your heart and lungs will be.

If you want to experiment with various swimming strokes, such as the breast stroke, you'll have to exercise different muscles. Since the breast stroke requires strong arms, shoulders, and chest you might initially work out with light weights. Don't overdo the weight training however, as this will make your muscles too stiff for swimming. Instead, try doing some of the water workouts mentioned earlier, such as chest pulls. These will work specifically on those muscles needed for the breast stroke.

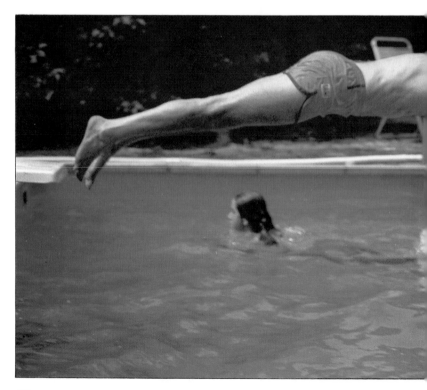

Another popular stroke is the backstroke, requiring powerful shoulders and back muscles. Standing in the water, leaning backward, and bringing your arms windmilling over your head will strengthen these muscles.

Since you propel yourself by using both your arms and your legs, don't forget to exercise the lower body. Try holding onto the edge of the pool and kicking your legs for a few minutes. The more often you do it, the easier it will become. You should also get into the habit of doing a few lunges, half-squats, and side bends during your workout routine. Since some strokes require you to scissor kick, it's also good for you to do a few minutes of these while holding onto the side of the pool. Some pools provide kick boards. Hold onto the board with your hands and then kick your way through a few laps.

Before you go swimming, it's advisable to stretch out on the side of the pool and limber up your muscles. Do a few toe touches and trunk twists. Arm circles get the shoulders loose. Since swimming is such a smooth, fluid motion, you want your body to be as loose as possible.

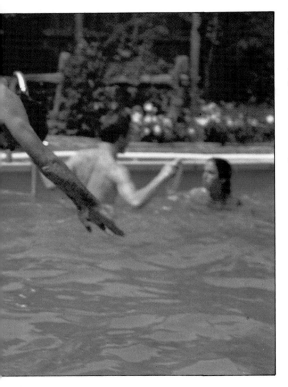

Swimming provides good exercise and is a convenient way of building up stamina and general cardiovascular fitness. Loosen up before you dive in and make sure the water is warm enough – getting into freezing cold water is dangerous and can be fatal.

▶ *JOGGING*

Of all sports, jogging has probably gotten the most attention over the past years. It seems that practically everyone has tried jogging. Unfortunately, some people try to overdo it at first and wind up injuring themselves. Jogging must be considered a sport that requires proper stretching and conditioning exercises.

Jogging requires a strong lower body and excellent cardiovascular development. Aerobics, swimming, and participation in other sports all increase the heart and lung capacity. Most experts agree that the best way to get involved with jogging is slowly. In the beginning, try just running in place for 4 minutes. You can even do this at home if you have a mat or other soft surface to absorb the pounding. After you've built up your running in place routine to 10 minutes, you can begin to jog outside. Keep in mind the word *jog*. You are not competing against anyone for speed. Take your time; find your own pace and rhythm. The more often you jog, the greater will be your endurance.

To make it easier and more fun, joggers should exercise to develop the leg muscles. Workouts in the swimming pool are ideal because they prevent any stress and yet provide great resistance to the movement of your muscles. Like isometrics where you press against an immovable object, working out in the water creates muscles.

You should also do an array of exercises to develop the abdomen, and tighten the waist. Side bends, trunk twists, and toe touches are all excellent for this. By coming up with your own exercise discipline, you'll be more likely to stick with it.

Once you have gotten into shape for jogging, you must remember to warm up each time you prepare to jog. Like any other sport, failure to warm up properly leads to injuries and then lack of interest in the exercise.

Spend a few minutes slowly jogging in place as you do a few neck rolls and shake out your arms. Then lean against a wall or tree and stretch out the leg tendons. Reach down and grasp your ankle, pulling your calf up close against the back of your thigh. Do this with each leg to limber up the lower leg. A few more minutes of shoulder shrugs and arm circles, a few deep breaths, and you're all set to hit the road!

Jogging is still the most popular sport and even though it is less strenuous than many other activities, you should warm up sensibly before starting.

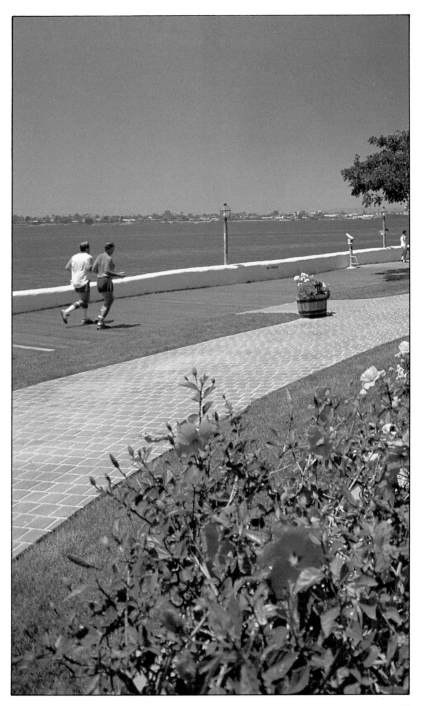

▶ FEET FIRST

In every sport — even those performed in the water — the feet play a vital role. From basketball to tennis, you can't make a move unless you use your feet. Since running is the choice of thousands of people, obviously attention must be paid to keeping the feet injury-free.

Read the section on selecting the right shoe and you'll see how complicated it can be to get the correct fit. But it's important — an incorrect choice of shoe and you may develop foot problems that might even need surgery to repair.

After you've selected the correct shoe, you should take the next important step — choosing where to run. Running on hard surfaces like city streets or even the beach may not be the smartest move. The more resistance the road's surface places on your pounding feet, the more shock ripples up your body. Constant pounding can injure the feet, legs, back, and even the abdomen, Some people believe that running on the beach is preferable, since at least you land on a soft surface. The beach, however, presents a different problem. Studies have shown that the normal jogging pattern of landing on your heels and rolling forward to your toes may cause injury to the Achilles tendon when jogging on the beach. Your heels dig so far down into the soft sand that thc tendon in the back of the ankle gets stretched too far. A constant stretching, on the average of 1,500 times every mile, can really put a strain on that tendon!

Another problem with running on city streets is the unpredictable nature of the surface. Holes, trash, even bumps may cause the foot to land unevenly. Anyone who has ever stepped in a hole can imagine the pain associated with unexpectedly landing in one when running.

Running through fields of grass may sound ideal, but there is always the chance that you'll step into a hole or on a rock, hurting your foot. Keep to surfaces that are relatively soft and easy to see.

The ideal surface to run on is the clay commonly found on oval tracks. Look at the various high schools in your neighborhood and see if there is such a track. If not, and if you don't mind running indoors, try to find a gymnasium that has a wood floor. Many of these floors are built on an "airspace" that has some give. The more flexibility on the surface, the less shock to your body.

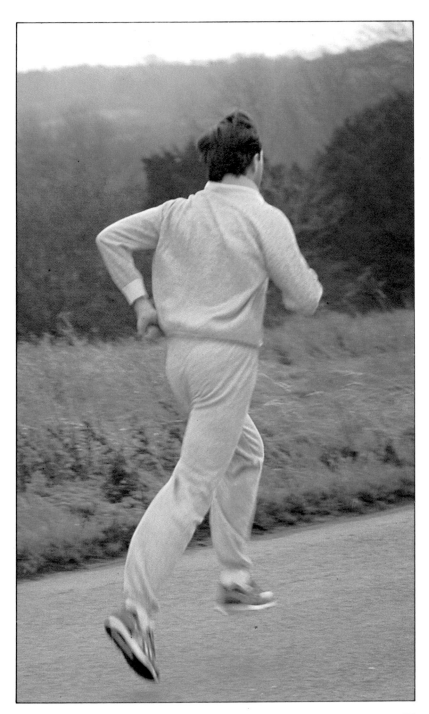

THE 20-MINUTE HOME WORKOUT

In our fast-paced world, some of us don't have the time to jog, play golf, or dribble a basketball. But that's no reason to stop exercising. If you can't get to a health club, let the health club come to you! Work out at home. Sometimes a home workout is even more enjoyable because you can listen to your favorite radio station or even watch television while you exercise.

Here's a simple exercise routine designed for the home. If you want to add new exercises to it, go right ahead. The more comfortable you are with your routine, the more you'll enjoy your healthy workout!

- Warm up by stretching your torso. Stand with feet apart, hands at your sides. Reach up with both arms and breathe in. Exhale and bring your arms down back to your sides. Repeat 5 times (5×).
- Spread your legs wide apart. Reach down with both your arms and clasp your left ankle. Hold for three seconds. Release and straighten up to the first position. Then repeat with your right ankle. Repeat 5×.
- Slowly jog in place on a cushioned mat for 6 minutes.
- With hands on hips, jump in place, alternately bending your knees and bringing them toward your chest. Continue for 2 minutes.
- Do 30 jumping jacks.
- Standing erect, bring your left elbow to your right knee; then bring your right elbow to your left knee. Repeat 30×.
- Still standing on the mat, pretend that you are jumping rope for 4 minutes.
- Lie on your back on the mat. With knees bent and arms extended through your legs, do 20 crunches by slowly raising your shoulders off the floor.
- Cool down by standing with your feet apart and hands at your sides. Breathe deeply as you raise your arms and circle them above your head. Exhale as your arms return to your sides. Continue for 2 minutes.

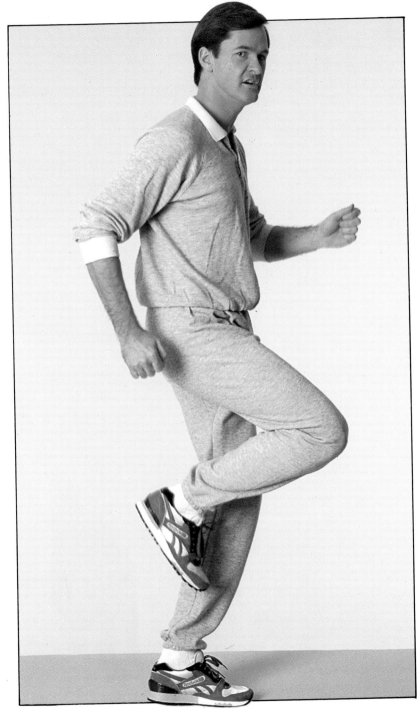

▶ THE DUMBBELL WORKOUT

By using a five-pound dumbbell (or an easy-to-hold five-pound object) you can increase the benefits of most aerobic workouts. The added weight puts more emphasis on the muscles of the upper body. Not only do you increase your heart and lung capacity and exercise the legs, you increase the muscle tone of your arms, shoulders, and chest!

Here are some recommended dumbbell workouts. Try them at your own pace.

ALTERNATE LIFTS

Holding the dumbbells by your sides, raise your left leg with knee bent. At the same time lift your right arm to your neck. Alternate with the right leg and left arm. Do 20 repetitions (20×).

DUMBBELL SWINGS

Stand still with legs apart at shoulder width. Hold both weights behind the left ear. Tighten the stomach muscles and twist around, swinging your hands in front of your face until the weights are behind the right ear. Repeat 30×.

DUMBBELL JOG

If you run regularly or are into aerobics, try this one. Slowly running in place, lift the left arm with the dumbbell as you lift your right leg. Repeat with the right arm and left leg as you jog in place for 3 minutes.

ALTERNATING FAST CURLS

Holding the dumbbells at your side with your palms facing forward, to fast curls, using alternating hands. Repeat 25× for each hand.

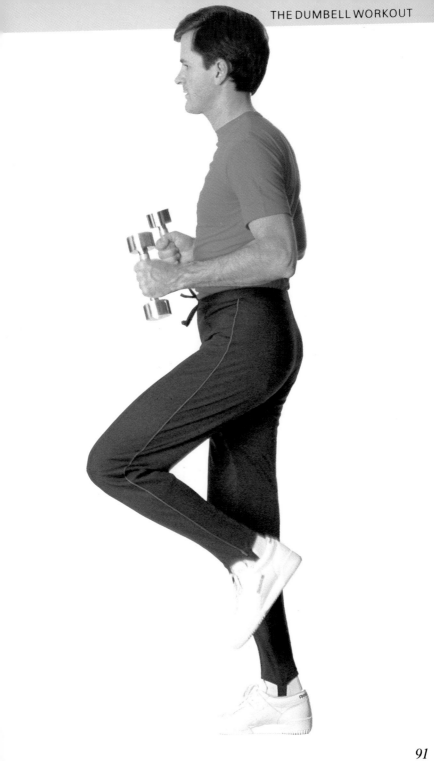

► THE BUSINESS TRIP WORKOUT

Staying out of town can really upset your daily routine. Eating in strange restaurants, sleeping in hotel rooms, even being without your favorite local newspaper — all can make you feel out of sorts. One way of keeping your sanity is to find time to continue your exercise workouts.

Here are some handy exercises that you can do in your hotel room while you're waiting for room service:

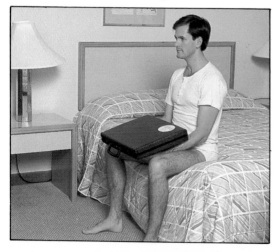

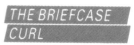
THE BRIEFCASE CURL

Since very few of us pack our dumbbells for a business trip, you have to improvise.

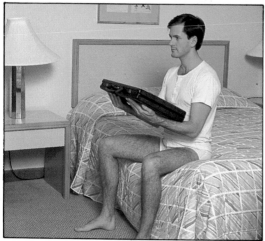

Sit on the desk chair or the edge of the bed. Grasp the briefcase.

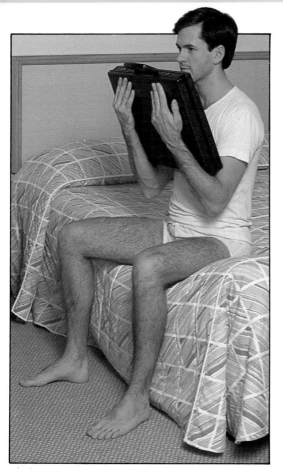

Then lift it, curling as you would a dumbbell. Do 20 repetitions (20×). If the briefcase is too light and you're accustomed to heavier weights, no problem. Try putting the Yellow Pages inside and then start curling, letting your fingers do the walking!

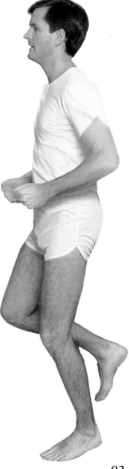

THE CARPET SHUFFLE

Since you probably didn't pack your jogging outfit, here's a way to run "on the run." Lock the door to your room. Probably your room contains the typically plush hotel carpeting, designed to keep the noise down. That carpeting will also absorb the shock as your feet dig in while you jog in place. You're all alone, so snap the television on to keep you company as you jog in your underwear, an experience you don't often get!

93

DOORWAY
PULL-UPS

Most hotel
doorways have some
sort of molding.
After warming up
with a few arm
circles and shoulder
shrugs, find a *secure*
molding over a
doorway in your
room.

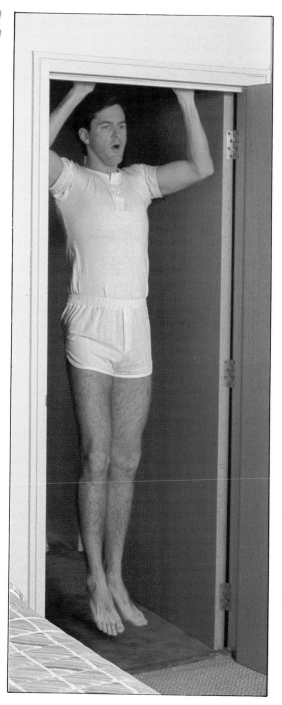

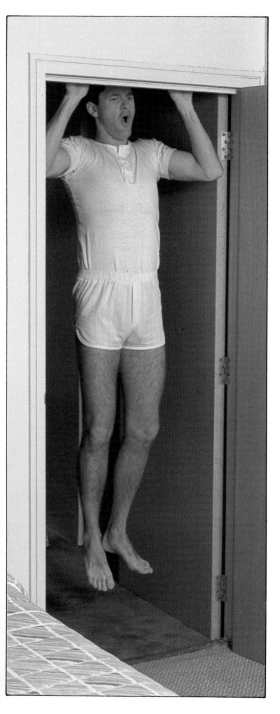

Test it by lifting yourself only inches from the floor. If it feels secure, do a few pull-ups.

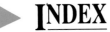